LOSE WEIGHT
WITHOUT MYSTERIES with
the PROGRESSIVE SWING DIET

Dr. D'Antoni's Progressive Slimming Method

Michele D'Antoni, MD

iUniverse, Inc.
New York   Bloomington

Lose Weight without Mysteries with the Progressive Swing Diet
Dr. D'Antoni's Progressive Slimming Method

iUniverse books may be ordered through booksellers or by contacting:

iUniverse
1663 Liberty Drive
Bloomington, IN 47403
www.iuniverse.com
1-800-Authors (1-800-288-4677)

Because of the dynamic nature of the Internet, any Web addresses or
links contained in this book may have changed since publication and
may no longer be valid. The views expressed in this work are solely those
of the author and do not necessarily reflect the views of the publisher,
and the publisher hereby disclaims any responsibility for them.

ISBN: 978-1-4401-4943-6 (pbk)
ISBN: 978-1-4401-4945-0 (cloth)
ISBN: 978-1-4401-4944-3 (ebk)

Printed in the United States of America

iUniverse rev. date: 7/1/2009

To my wife Valeria With love

*"Obesity is not a sweet cradle,
but a crumbling alcove,
where it is possible
to escape from,
thanks to our intelligence, shrewdness
and will"*

Michele D'Antoni, M. D.
Web site: www.micheledantoni.it

Preface

Today food science is a topic of great interest: "we are what we eat" and therefore, as a consequence, not only the quantity but also the quality of food.

In particular, some "fitness" models are those of a perfect balance between weight and height. It is hardly possible with a continuous proposal of particular diets and with the possibility of eating titbit. Probably, everybody eats greedily probably to forget an atavic hunger.

It is obvious therefore that there is the need of slimming diets to make up for food excess and it is a particular merit of Dr. D'Antoni to write "losing weight with the Progressive Method".

At last we give importance to the dynamic action specific of food and to the fact that the food intake is not directly proportional to the anabolism, that is accumulation of matter and energy. You can eat a lot and eliminate the same and inversely you can eat little and absorb everything: <u>blessed diencephalic set point</u>. It is the regulator of metabolism positioned in the central nervous system, above the hypophysis, strictly connected with nervous fibers and hormones.

Beyond all-out viewpoints that, sometimes, conquer a space on mass-media, the debate on diets reveals deep ethical implications related to the right of free choice which should characterize all the protective measures about health or personal integrity. This principle which is certainly right could extend also to the refusal of the laws punishing as crime the personal use of crash helmets and seat belts. The question is undoubtedly fascinating. It is certainly true that who gets an illness or an injury, damages all the society indirectly, both from an economic point of view and as to the relations for all the citizens, but it would be however dangerous to grant the State the paternalistic power to decide what is good or what is bad for all citizens. Following this principle, in fact, we would end up with the prohibition of cigarettes, high-proof spirits, or even to rationate the hours dedicated to television like parents do with their children.

We have to say, however, as we will see better later, that diets have their specific features. It is not a choice involving benefits and risks only for those who follow them, but also for the whole community.

In addition, in the field of diets aimed, for example, at the growth of young, that is when assimilation prevails on disassimilation, the decision is not taken by the direct interested party but by his parents. As we all know, in a state of right, parents could always be deprived of their parental authority from the state when they do not protect their children in an adequate way.

Since we are almost concluding this foreword, it is necessary to draw some conclusions, that considered the actual animated debate about diets, do not pretend to be considered conclusions but rather to highlight some aspects.

The first is that, today the decrease of infectious diseases in our country risks to favor a certain snobbish "distance" from the quality of food, seen as the heritage of a period already almost completely concluded. It is not like this. And if you do not want to take a sort of evolutionistic vision into consideration, we have to overcome the logic of automatism of preservation and find in the nutritional intervention the real dimension of the care of life in all its stages and forms. From the other side the food intervention must never lose its targeted character. Therefore, the adequate administration is not an end in itself but always supports the welfare of a single person and the society he belongs to.

This means that the intervention has always a personal and individual character and a social valency. This assumption, mostly implicit, must not be forgotten. The meaning of a right nutrition with the production also of antibodies consists in the worry of the safeguard of social welfare, compared to the eventual epidemiological risks. The consequence is the public intervention regulated by appropriated legislative forms. If this can result marginal, I think that you have to highlight, in the first place, the ethical-anthropological feature of the legislative intervention which can only on this basis legislate about the compulsoriness of food and drugs' control specially made.

As to these reflections of social contract, we have also to take the public ethics into consideration, as well as the relationship between risks and benefits. However, they have to place itself in the viewpoint of the whole public health, which is the only reference point.

Of course a deep work like this one by Michele D'Antoni, for its detailed organization, supplies the reader with extension of the subject and the pleasure and burden of food. Therefore this work will be able to give advice about the search of best food trends in an active way.

Chief dvsn Virology
D. Cotugno Hospital
In Naples - Italy
President of Italian
Society of Immuno-Oncology
Project dir. Nat. cancer Inst.
Bethesda. Md. 1971/75
Member of International
Academy of United Nations

Contents

Second Part
OBESITY TODAY

Third Part
LOSE WEIGHT EASILY AND GET RID OF DIET ADDICTION

Fourth Part
ILLUSTRATION AND EXPLANATION OF THE PROGRESSIVE METHOD

Fifth Part
A GOOD EXAMPLE OF HEALTY DIET EVEN FOR THOSE WHO DO NOT HAVE TO LOSE WEIGHT

Technical section

Welcome to the readers

The author hopes that all the scientific contents
of this book are fully understood.
We have done our best to disclose
to the readers elementary concepts
of Food Science, by informing them
in detail and soundness,
counting on their cleverness and
assessment.

Notice For The Readers

What is the fundamental mechanism, which allows keeping the body weight uniform

Food Science teaches us that any organism needs a certain amount of daily calories to perform its own vital functions. This calorie requirement can largely vary depending on a great number of factors. The most important are: sex, weight, height, age, build and life style. An adult of 70 Kg dealing with clerical work, needs about 2400 daily calories1, that is 35 cal/Kg a day. They are divided into the following optimal proportion:

CARBOHYDRATES (sugars): 380 g, multiplied by 4 cal/g is 1520 calories, equal to 63%; PROTIDS (proteins): 70 g, multiplied by 4 cal/g is 280 calories, equal to 11%;

LIPIDS (fats): 70 g, multiplied by 9 cal/g is 630 calories, equal to 26%;

Of course, this proportion is applicable to people in perfect metabolic efficiency with the same bony structure and daily physical exertion.

If we introduce more calories than our daily requirement, the complicated neuro-hormonal system controlling the body weight (the so-called set-point by American dieticians) makes them discharge, within certain limits, increasing metabolic exchanges.

Vice versa, if we introduce less calories than our requirement, the metabolic rhythm is slackened in order to conform to the energy introduced, within certain limits, too. The metabolic slackening plays essentially a protective role and it has been handed down genetically by our ancestors. In ancient times, in fact, their bodies had to cope with hard environmental conditions, such as lack of food, famines and so on. It seems that western industrialized peoples (Europe, USA, etc.) waste food, introducing daily about 1000 calories each more than necessary for maintaining their weight. These calories are generally almost burnt up by our

---

1   For the woman, always for a very light physical activity during the whole 24 hours, the value, compared to that of man, would reduce by about 10-11%. For both sexes, the metabolic efficiency and the consumption of calories/Kg of bodily weight are considered inversely proportional to weight (see explanatory chart page 6), Metabolism in obese or overweight people show, moreover, a considerable slackening. This makes inconceivable, even for young patients but with very low consumptions of energy, the consumption of food levels superior to 30-35 cal/Kg of bodily weight (woman-man). We have constantly referred to this value for the whole treatise.

body, thus increasing the amount of metabolic exchange. A few people only start putting weight on, just because the do not burn them up. On the contrary, as to commonplace, if you put on weight "because you eat more than necessary", all western peoples, except some rare exception, should in the long run put on dozens and dozens of kilos progressively.

It is not necessary to get rid of these daily extra 1000 calories to make someone lose weight, since with a minor food intake, our body reacts by lowering its metabolic rhythm. Therefore, in such a case, after losing 1-2 kg your weight will become stable. If you want to lose more, you will have to follow a low caloric diet, that is with less calories than those you need. When we have saved a total of 6000 calories (or 7000 according to others), we will notice the loss of the first kilo.

This happens to normal patients, introducing more than 1000 extra daily calories. If this surplus would not have been introduced and therefore the patients would follow a strict diet, their body, already used to lower its metabolic needs, will suffer less from further restrictions.

Well, if these elementary and basic notions would be taught when you attend secondary school (if better elementary school) we will have far fewer obese people, and these will be able to cope with their problem better.

Just think that, instead, in Italy everybody knows how an internal combustion engine works (only because they studied it at the driving test). Many people even know how to calculate the consumption of their car, horsepower, usage, etc.!

RANGE VALUES HUMAN ENERGETIC REQUIREMENT			
	Kg Weight	Daily calories	CAL./Kg
WOMAN	55	1850	33,7
LIGHT	60	1960	32,6
ACTIVITY	65	2060	31,6
	70	2165	30,9
MAN	60	2250	37,5
LIGHT	65	2360	36,3
ACTIVITY	70	2465	35,2
	75	2575	34,3
	80	2680	33,5
	85	2790	32,8

For both sexes, the metabolic efficiency and the consumption of calories/kg of bodily weight must be considered, from my personal reflection, inversely proportional to weight (see explanatory chart)

What are the most serious mistakes you make when you start a slimming diet?

- *Considering important only the amount of kilos to lose, while the mistake is underestimating the way in which you lose them (see fundamental scheme on page 43) because a result, which apparently could be important, is absolutely insignificant with a close examination.*
- *Thinking that a single diet, even if well-structured, can make lose on its own and identically repeated all necessary kilos. That is why the Progressive Method fills at last the most serious gap in slimming treatments, that is the absolute need of a continuous variation of diets to reach the aim.*
- *Cutting off carbohydrates and supply oneself with sugars in sweets.*
- *Thinking that you have to lose perhaps many kilos, when on the contrary you often need to lose a few, but in the right parts.*
- *Feeling attraction for all what seems eccentric and bizarre (crazy diets, liquid food, fasting, laxative herbs, yoga, hypnosis, etc.) even if this is in clear contrast with the most elementary rules of medicine.*
- *Starting straightaway with too drastic diets (you can lose much weight at the beginning but not later) or too easy ones (with the risk of becoming chronic, a fundamental concept never so far tackled and pointed out by any author).1*
- *Thinking of the existence of people who knows mysterious ways out from obesity (which must not involve food sacrifice, calorie counting, use of scales!).*
- *These are the reasons why, in the world, some diets including everything but carbohydrates and sugars are often successful. People who do not want to include them think they are responsible for their same transformation into fats and therefore into pads.*
- *This diet (or better this illusion), like comets, is followed cyclically every 5-10 years in Europe, allowing everybody to lose weight by eating as much as one likes any food but carbohydrates (that therefore in percentage would be reduced from 55-60% to zero).*

---

1   The lack of a guide and a precise program, in the short or long run, has provoked the creation of a real crowd of stragglers (by tens million in Europe).

The human body will therefore be subject to a huge chemical work against nature, because the organism must synthesize the lack of glicids starting from fats and proteins introduced with no limit. The few kilos lost, moreover, are those from a loss of water which the body had to get rid of more than usual to discharge the protein charge (enormous in some cases).

In Italy, apart from the deviation of metabolism because of the change in the diet, had been introduced into the diet, very expensive tablets taken together (such as diuretics, laxatives, thyroid hormones, amphetamine).

In addition, you have to take at least 6-8 a day!

It is pretty sure, in comparison, that the "great dilemma" about the use of anorectics (see page 23) which we have faced in a scrupulous way is a child's play, a real marginal problem. [2]

---

2   The Health Department on February 10th 1997, has forbidden in Italy the sale and the manufacturing, from chemist's, of these kind of drugs based on galenic products, setting free the sale of products from pharmaceutical industries containing a drug by time, and in addition, with the prescription within the box.

What are the main *"it is not true"* questions to remove at once?

- Diet is a synonym of slimming treatment: in the last one, in fact, it is comprehended also the concept of guide and global strategy, lacking to the single diet.
- The dietician must only weigh people and check their arterial pressure: they must be an attentive guide, clever, always looking for the right way for their patient.
- Keeping always the right weight means to be for your entire life on diet: in this book we say just the opposite.
- The so-called "blood test", even more accurate, are able to clear up all kinds of obesity.
- Slimming drugs do exist. We can rather say we can use drugs during slimming treatment (and it is not the same).
- The human chorionic gonadotropin (HCG) is a slimming drug: vice versa it is a tonic.
- Just with pasta and carbohydrates nobody puts on weight unless they eat more than one kilo a day (see African people and Third World).
- People with blood pressure inferior to 100 mm Hg cannot be on diet: generally speaking, by introducing more proteins, the pressure value gets back to normal better than injecting whole boxes of surrenal cortex.
- People suffering from nervous breakdown: a new figure often improves their mood better than a drawer full of tranquilizers.
- People playing a lot of sport lose weight better than others: the failure is a matter of topical interest because these people, keep on their favourite sport, when they get home they intake more calories than the amount they spent practicing sport.
- A slimming diet works better if the patient is educated or has some knowledge in the field: these people assume that they are able to follow a diet by themselves.
- They will never lose more than 2-3 kg and they will spend their entire life to discuss about diets in drawing-rooms, in offices, while others, that probably do not understand a lot, follow the advice of a dietician and in the meantime obtain the ideal weight.

- There is only a diet, even if personalized and well-individualized, able by itself to make a given patient lose weight. The planning of the Progressive Method fills a gap which is always involved in the strategy of slimming treatment, that is the lack of a systematic dietetic program which is absolutely necessary to get the result.
- Patients who can discuss with a psychologist during the treatment lose weight better. In this case, patients will be tempted to abandon, at least temporary, the slimming cycle to settle their unconscious. Who has not existential problems? In obese people, speaking too much is a good excuse not to lose weight.

What I ask my patients, on the contrary, is to awake their sleepy will, the true and real one, with no negotiation with the themselves, getting out from the psychological lethargy, trying to conquer again themselves, their lost ground, their missed opportunity. At most, by using some tiny shrewdness, as my motto says at the beginning of this book. If you experience a weakness, it is better to look at it with cleverness, with the viewpoint of maturity and complete recovery of personality which could not be too late. Dietician's help will be fundamental to get this goal.

FIRST PART

THE MAIN MISUNDERSTANDINGS ABOUT SLIMMING DIET

What should be the role of the dietician in the planning and in the conduct of the treatment?

Since the first years of the XX century we can find remarkable collections in every language, where physicians and others indulge their fancy in listing, in order to lose weight, nutritious food with few fats, selected in order to satisfy even the pretension of the most refined palates.

What is the reason why nobody succeeds, with some good will and by consulting one of these books, in finishing a considerable loss of weight superior to the famous limit of 2-3 kg?

The explanation is very simple; by following these diets people do succeed in losing some weight. Everybody knows that eating less than necessary, every organism must inexorably lose some kilos.

What you never succeed in obtaining, on the contrary, is to finish the whole slimming treatment.

The way to the goal is comparable to a steep mountain path which few expert guides know well and which gets through a real jungle of risks. Contrary to what you expect, they always lie in wait when you get much closer to the end. For example, patients weighing 90 kg who want to reach 75, by following always the same diet described on one of these books or on a fashion magazine, will succeed in reaching probably with ease 87 kg or even 86 in a short time, say 20-30 days, but they will never succeed on their own, by repeating mechanically the same diet, to follow the next steps, that is from 86 to 75. If they should reach this goal, it is pretty difficult they make some mistakes, which will lead them astray.

The dietician must not be therefore only a physician prescribing drastic diets (steak and salad without dressing) or suggesting succulent low calorie recipes during a consultation behind his desk, according to his personal guidance. Vice versa, having a wide experience in the field, he must organize the treatment and outline with charisma a strategy for his patients for the whole treatment they have to follow.

What is the difference between slimming diet and slimming treatment?

Even if these two words may appear as synonym, they are two concepts completely different. Our times, which pretend to be based on clearness, sometimes tend to confuse and distort too many things, included these two terms. For diet we mean a therapeutic treatment used by a health operator to cure not only obesity and thinness, but also many other unhealthy conditions of great importance for human pathology: if you follow an appropriate diet, a great number of disease of the digestive system (gastritis, duodenitis, ulcers, colitis, degenerative diseases of liver, of pancreas, of bile ducts; not to mention arteriosclerosis, all kinds of cardiopathy and kidney diseases) are capable of substantial improvement. All these unhealthy conditions which may be more or less severe, have in common the fact that, if they are treated in the very first stage, they can improve and frequently also stop. This will happen if the patients are able to create an inversion of tendency of their metabolism by following a healthy diet.

As you can notice, so far we have spoken about diet without even mentioning slimming treatment. That is, we have examined a series of organs and systems whose functions can be influenced by the assumption of a certain type of diet. *Therefore, diet means simply a particular way of eating:* following a diet does not imply following a slimming treatment. In fact, a slimming treatment can involve that of a diet, but eventually could do without it. You could, for example, lose some weight by doing an intense physical activity, or following intense pharmacological treatment, without modifying your food habits at all.

Unfortunately, generally speaking, these possibilities become theoretical and it always happens that you have to follow a diet; that is why, in this medical sector, the two terms have become by mistake synonyms.

Which is the real identikit of obese or overweight subjects? Gourmets or "non-gourmets"? Misinformed or in bad faith?

- They persist in limiting carbohydrates (pasta, rice, bread, pulses) or even abolishing them. With unbelievable naivety (bordering bad faith), he ignores that the real problems are cheese, salami and cold pork meats, oil, salt, sweets and generally all the food containing plenty of fats and sugars.
- Instead of savoring genuine tastes typical of every food, or trying to exalting particular flavorings or fragrances, they do their best to cover tastes, adding to each course plenty of salt and oil. At the end, we can consider them rather "non-gourmets" than gourmets. If somebody should not believe what I am saying, just try sprinkling salt or oil everywhere. He will understand that all the tastes of the different vegetables (carrots, eggplants, tomatoes, and so on) and of meat (chicken, rabbit, beef and so on) will taste all the same.
- Very often, the obeses have entered on their passive many negative experiences. They do not speak about them, as you would expect, and show no disappointment regarding themselves (maybe they have to reproach themselves with scarce will and lack of perseverance) or the operator who has led these vain attempts.

This surprising passive attitude is revealed also in those cases in which the patients, improving its degree of information, have understood which mistakes have been made towards them.

They understood, for example, that the first time they were given massive doses of drugs to ease hunger, and the subsequent slimming was caused only by a loss of appetite. In the following attempt, the few kilos of weight were lost thanks to a very drastic diet; in another one, for example, a certain success was obtained thanks to a long prolongation of the treatment.

An explanation of the reason why in this field people accept everything philosophically and patiently could be that obeses have never a clear conscience. For their daily breaking the rules and diets they have not the nerve to invest anybody with a responsibility.

Have a try. Invite at your place obese people and do not give them anything to eat, maybe on the pretext there is any gas to cook. Convince them to drink plenty of water, even exalting the freshness, savor and so on. The following day when they will notice inevitably, weighing themselves, to have lost even half a kilo, instead of thinking they lost weight because they skipped a meal reluctantly, they would become convinced that, with a probability of 60-70% some water with "dietetic powers" flow from you pipes.

When they will tell somebody, many undoubtedly will laugh at them. Some others, do not be surprised, will take them seriously. Probably you will receive some calls from somebody asking for a bottle of your water, which has proved so precious.

This may sound a paradox or even exaggerated but can happen. The obeses are from one side bombarded by messages expressed in bad faith and from the other one, such messages have always clung them to the following great illusion. There must be a "magic" shortcut, a "secret" as big as probably very banal. The official medicine has never thought about, by sheer coincidence, and however - this is obvious - has nothing to do with calorie counting and food control!

What are the main explanations given until today about the origin of obesity? The mystery is clearing up at last.

Beyond the complex and sometimes too different classifications proposed by uncountable scholars, for the purposes of our illustrative treatise, we will deal with *two fundamental types of obesity*. The first is the *endogenic* or *endocrinic* one, which is caused by a glandular block (hypophysis, ovaries, thyroid, pancreas, suprarenal cortex, Fröhlich and so on). The second one called *exogenic* (we will explain later why) is caused by an exaggerated food quantity.

Very few are the real forms caused by glandular block: subjecting hundred obese people to the most sophisticated hormonal dosage, only 1 or 2% show alterations which can explain why somebody has become an obese person.

The other, the exogenic one, generally considered the principal, is based on the concept of overfeeding and should be explained in depth. In fact, we cannot explain why, after all, few people are obese if we reflect on the fact that most western peoples eat much more than necessary. If it would be enough to eat a lot to become obese automatically, everybody should be obese. In reality, according to the Italian statistics, only one people out of ten is obese. Therefore, even this form of obesity has to be connected to the first group because it has on its basis a mechanism of jamming which is luckily absent in the majority of organisms.

According to a statistic reliable enough, in fact, Italians (but the average is common to all western nations) swallow daily about 1000 calories more than their food requirements. Now then, if a normal person swallowed 6000 calories (or 7000, according to others), he would put on 1 kg. If the indiscriminate statement were true, in other words that you become obese only because you eat more than necessary, every person should put on one kilo every 6 days, and therefore 5 kilos a month (and 60 a year)! Of course, this will happen to all the peoples who enjoy an affluent welfare.

This is not true, as most recent acquisitions about the subject have proved. In fact, in a part of our brain called diencephalon, we can find a nerve center responsible for the maintenance of weight (*set-point* of the American authors:

the first to use this concept, it seems it was Nisbett R.E. in 1972 - even if he himself in his scientific work, says he was influenced by his colleagues Cabanac, Duclaux and Spector)[1]. Practically, in the greatest part of human beings it always works very well. Its task is to make excess calories burn. When vice versa calories are not enough, it makes them be sufficient by lowering the level of metabolism. In conclusion, it is then correct to say that only few people, among those who eat a lot, put on weight.

And after all their nerve center does work perhaps at 95-97% instead than 100%, being already this slight anomaly enough to have a tendency to put on or lose weight.

In fact, if the deficit of working were greater, an overeating patient, in short time would certainly put on dozens and dozens of kilos, instead of the few ones that generally a normal obese person puts on. Without considering that, in these cases, nature sets limits beyond which, luckily, only very rare cases arrive at. For their exceptionality, in fact, they are written in the pages of worldwide newspapers.

By deficit of working of this center, we mean, in this treatise, the would-be use of excess calories from some organisms which form the adipose deposits.

---

1   By *set-point,* beyond the simple literary meaning of "regulating level", we mean in this book, a regulating center or cerebral thermostat. We suppose, in fact, that, even if it is situated inside the central nerve system, it may consist in a delicate system control of the body weight, through the constant regulation of adipose deposit in the organism. It elaborates, probably in continues contact with more endocrine glands, biochemical messages (coming from the periphery through the haematic flow) and transmits in return orders to the adipose cells. We have sometimes believed to be able to explain the reasons of its malfunctioning with some of the remarkable scientific discoveries (impossibility of adequate use of thyroid hormones from obese people, hyper-insulin intolerance, hypo-thalamic lesions, enzymatic defect, deficit from brown adipose tissue, adipose heredity and so on). All the same no recent explanation put forward is completely convincing and the problem of its functioning is still open. Last most recent discovery is that of leptin or adipsin, a hormonal substance (protein) which conveys biochemical messages from adipose deposit to the hypothalamic *set-point* (cerebral). Its lack provokes in rats stocks of obese families (ob-ob) which can go back to their normal condition after its administra-tion. As to men, on the contrary, the expectations have been disappointed since in obese people this substance is present at levels even greater than the normal ones, and we do not succeed in understanding why it does not work provoking the loss of weight. We suppose it could be a problem of "receptorial deafness", that is to locate the places, the receptors, where the hormone should bind itself ("Il Giornale del Medico", November 28, 1996). Not to mention that (and this is my personal theory) these biochemical receptors could also be totally absent among very obese people, and only partially present in the moderate obesity. In such a case, the problem would be already definitely solved. If our genome has not created receptors, we could do nothing to create them by ourselves; and the level of leptin, from its side, even if elevated with hormone administration, would not produce any effect on obesity as it would not have no place where to bind itself chemically.

In short, these people become obese because they do not succeed, food being equal, in dissipating the same quantities of energy than normal subjects do[2].

Anyway, we can observe more severe cases (all those who have made uncountable attempts, especially woman) where this situation of scarce or very scarce use of calories introduced takes place unfortunately also when the subjects follow a diet properly related to their weight[3]. For this reason, many experts, included myself, can quite confirm that this complex nerve structure (set-point) must be necessarily connected to the fat cells. In fact, it has a strict conservative-like control over the adipose tissue. However, if you succeed in losing weight according to the Progressive Method, because of the action of bewilderment that the continuous variation of calories introduced seems to exercise on the center of hunger and on the diencephalic centers, as a consequence, a "normalization" of this nerve center will take place[4].

In fact, as results from the vast number of patients treated in my office during 20 years of activity, the general average of patients who have concluded a treatment according to our criteria (Progressive Method) have maintained easily their new weight, following diets foreseen at various caloric levels.

---

2   However, if an obese person did not introduce such surplus (or exceeding quantity) normally, he would only be potentially obese, as predisposed subject. Such a concept cannot be exploited in practice, even if it is of great importance. Nobody in fact will set restrictions on food, and in addition during childhood, for fear of being a subject predisposed to obesity. However, conclusions of studies into children adopted in Denmark from 1924 to 1947, conducted by Stunkard, have demonstrated the possibility to inherit a predisposition to obesity. On the other side, other former studies by the same author (Goldblatt, Moore, Stunkard, 1964, Jama; Stunkard and coll., 1972, Jama) and further surveys into women from different social classes conducted in New York by other scholars, have demonstrated what follows. Subjects belonging to lower classes were stricken by obesity statistically speaking, six times more in comparison with those belonging to upper classes, who probably had a better food education. Do not forget, however, that many people become obese even if they had not inherited any genetic predisposition, having the research on their family tree tested negative. If you consider that for some people the tendency to put on weight starts when they are children or adolescents, many others become obese only after 25 years, or all of a sudden, at any age, after a psychic shock. In all the cases, the final effect consists, therefore, in the defective attitude of the *set-point*, which does not succeed in burning excess calories. This happens either way people have inherited a certain genetic predisposition to obesity or not.

3   Practically it seems that all these (mainly a crowd of women but men too) had lost their "right" to introduce their daily calories.

4   By normalization of set-point I mean not only the possibility to maintain, after the course, the new weight by adapting the right diets (see page 56), but also a major resistance, different from one to another, to put on weight after repeated events of big nourishment. All those patients confirmed that after any preceding diet never before they had had this benefit. This normalization includes also a preservation of appetite within a range closer to normality, diminishing or also disappearing in some subjects the enormous compulsiveness towards food.

The nerve central system plays an important role in the metabolism of the adipose tissue. This happens through sophisticated hormonal functions and basic mechanism of reply to environmental stimulus such as control of body temperature, food intake, general water balance, arterial pressure, emotions, stress and so on. The firm belief that the principal regulating mechanisms of body weight would be found within the central nerve system derives, on the other hand, from elementary considerations, too.

I have also noted on the basis of numerous personal observations, even outside my usual activity, that a psychic shock has very often caused many people to lose weight. Before they had made great efforts to lose weight, while within the same family, some components, who seemed to stay slim for all life long, started putting on weight, *though they were always been heavy eaters.*

We can say then that a psychic shock can suddenly provoke obesity or thinness in subjects who follow their usual diet, because the biochemical messages so far produced by *set-point* are disturbed. This is a proof that this weight control system is inside our brain and that the *set-point,* even if it exercises on obese people a conservative-like control over their metabolism, has nothing to do with genetic heredity and must not be confused with it.

It is of course very unlikely that a violent prolonged psychic stress (or a single shock too) can provoke the change of a genetic asset already settled in an obese subject. Vice versa, emotional-like events can influence very well a system of weight control situated inside our brain, whose regulating point, either way right or wrong, has been created after we were born.

Therefore, if from one side, the *set-point* cannot ignore the genetic message, from the other part, it modulates its own regulating point according to the environmental situation of a given organism in the development of its own vital cycle. Even severe cranial shocks with hospitalization for loss of conscience have shown, a couple of months after the accidents, the development of obesity in subject always long-limbed. On the contrary, sudden thinness in subjects always obese (less frequent eventuality).

From these last considerations, we can deduce that the *set-point* is located in the cranium (hypothalamus), with the danger, that if this is banged, well, it can break down, too! Other recent acquisitions have drawn attention to the so-called brown adipose tissue, a particular kind of adipose tissue, which seems to be located preferentially around the skeleton.

This tissue seems supervising the very delicate function of thermogenesis, that is dissipation of energy. Therefore, we have supposed that from its deficit it can derive the incomplete removal of excess calories. Some others, still, have stated that the diencephalic nerve center modulates its own working and its own regulating point in strict connection with this adipose organ.

Nevertheless, I do not think right, in this treatise, to go into a question, which still needs some other confirmations[5].

---

5   Z. Glick, G. Brag, *Brown Adipose Tissue: Thermic Response Increased by a Single Low Protein, High Carbohydrate Meal,* "Science", 213, 1125 (1982); P. V. Sukhatieme and S. Margen, *Autoregulatory Homeostatic Nature of Energy Balance,* Amer. J. Clinical Nur., 35, 355 (1982).

What are the main drugs used in the obesity treatment? The "great dilemma" of hunger-repressing drugs

Certainly, one of the most discouraging aspect of obesity is that, while there is a cause for most disease and after you detect it you can propose a proper drug, on the contrary for obesity is different. Nevertheless the most accurate analysis, it is very unusual to find a precise cause and consequently, hardly ever you can propose a resolutory drug, that is a slimming one.

Even if detoxifying drugs are not meant for the treatment of obesity, they have proved particularly useful because they have a general tonic effect on our organism. In addition they restore the liver function and exercise a favorable action on fat metabolism, therefore setting in motion the lipids in excess and lowering the cholesterol levels. Personally, I have used them successfully in patients with hepatic problems, dyslipidosis, who had followed very strict slimming diets.

***

The same substances exercise actions clinically appreciable on the central nervous system, on memory, preserving in general cellular membranes of the whole organism. But we cannot consider them slimming drugs.

On the contrary, in everybody's cast of mind - except the experts - the concept that slimming drugs do exist is deep-rooted.

The truth is that a usual and sensational misunderstanding has been created about it, and since ever it has characterized the field of slimming diets.

If there were a category of drugs capable to treat obesity, we should notice that, maintaining and not modifying at all our food habits, when we take the drug we should have a loss of weight. Unfortunately today we have no category of drugs capable to give this result, unless, in the same time, the patients follow a slower calorie diet than their requirement.

Having made these preliminary remarks, it is worth speaking about some drugs which can be used during a slimming treatment. Of course, it would be better not to need them at all, even if they could be of help in particular difficult moments.

I refer to the activators of metabolism (thyroid hormones and iodated compound) and anorectics[1].

As to the first, we have to say that today they have almost been abandoned. In fact, the great part of slimming provoked by them is related to the so-called slim mass (muscles) that has nothing to do with fat.

Anorectics, notwithstanding the ferocious criticism against them, represent sometimes the only remedy capable to save a treatment. Even if the dietician and the patient conduct the treatment in an impeccable way, it is possible that an impressive pang of hunger jeopardizes it, making the whole progress so far vain. This sort of drug can be therefore precious to overcome these possible periods of crisis. The continuous use for months or years is literally inconceivable, if it is the main element of the treatment, because in the long run it may prove treacherous.

From my personal experience, and many colleagues, it seems that during prolonged assumption, not only the hunger becomes weaker, but the whole organism probably tends to absorb fewer fats than usual.

Afterwards, by interrupting its administration, even if the patients will manage to calm their appetite, the intestine will absorb much more fats that those absorbed during its administration. Not to mention, then, the further complications arising in the relationship with patients. Considered that there are subjects (about 10%) who do not bear the drug[2], it will be necessary to alert one by one, since it may be possible that you do chance, without your knowledge, upon the intolerant subject.

Therefore it is advisable to explain in details all the symptoms that could be establish a connection with the assumption of tablets. This is to avoid that, by continuing the assumption, some trouble are always more evident day after day and the patients will be obliged to see their doctor.

Sometimes, some dramatic misunderstandings can also happen. For example, some disorders related to the assumption of these drugs from patients absolutely refractory to them (if they would have been warned about the side

---

1   In this book, we mean by "anorectics" only the drugs which were very trendy in Italy in the last decades, mostly based on molecules called dietil-propione, fendimetrazina, etc. Therefore the pharmacological associations, mainly of the galenic type, are not included. These last ones are prepared by pharmacologists under medical prescription and they were at long last abolished by the Health Ministry on 10 February 1997. In addition, they were very expensive and they were extensively used in Italy in the last years, before their cutting out.

2   Average mean emerging from the collection of clinical news of patients, during the stories of the slimming treatment followed before.

effects, they would have interrupted at once the assumption) are interpreted as symptoms of serious illness.

For these reasons, more than for the other ones (more subtle and often even unknown by the same experts) related to the rebound of appetite and absorption of fats, many patients interrupt the assumption after having used them for a long time, (more than 2-3 months).

As you can assume, the problem would be easily solved with a lot of good will and detailed and more correct information.

Anorectics, therefore, are condemned fiercely for a reason which would be definitely surmountable, that is, as we have already said, that of undesirable reactions from patients intolerant to the drug who are not informed in details.

Instead, the greater harm escapes the majority (the experts, too) and consists in the rebounce of weight and appetite after an assumption prolonged for years. In these cases, by interrupting them, metabolism will slow down considerably. For this event, instead, there is nothing to do. The danger of tolerance and addiction to these drugs is very overestimated. In my long enough career of dietician, in fact, I have never chanced upon stories of normal patients (except 1 or 2 cases) that, after the assumption of regular doses of anorectics for one, two or even three months, they were addicted against their will. These events, instead, like others of the same kind (alcoholism, etc.), are almost always localized to extreme cases[3].

Of course, it is also necessary to put oneself in the doctor's place whom patients often conceal the slimming treatment because they are afraid to be disapproved. Some doctors, not knowing at all about the assumption of tablets, run into certain patients who seem to develop a somehow indecipherable, mysterious and serious pathology. For example: some sudden cephalea which increases more and more every day (and when they take a table); or inexplicable throbbing in quiet patients, or still tremors in the hands and insomnia. Obviously these patients are part of the about 10% of subjects allergic to the drug.

Further uneasiness consists in the unpleasant surprise the party concerned get as soon as they start reading the instructions contained in the inner sheet of the box.

Generally the pharmaceutical industries producing these products, include long lists of side effects and complications which can occur. The reason is that they got stung by the misuse of the past and, in the light of the recent ministerial rules, they maybe got tired to be indirectly touched by the

---

3   I reassert again the conviction that these are always extreme cases, and that, for example in my long career, I have ever seen developing in the relationship with my patients who had taken them before.

problem of anorexia. On the other side, the patients will be depressed if they ask advice in their circle of friends. With a 10% of intolerant patients, it will be very easy to run into people who will strongly advise them against their use. This is very common because these people were not warned about these drugs and since they were refractory, they had had very negative experiences. But even this is not right! Who is asking could belong to the 90% that bears this drug well. Perhaps, in this case, it could be precious to make them overcome some critical moment[4].

What is then the solution of the "great dilemma"? To use or not to use anorectics? Would not it be better to listen to whom proposes for some time to cancel them from the lists of drugs? In fact, considering the potential dangerousness and the scarce individual responsibility, which could totally lack, the patient could take the way to anorexia.

Of course, their striking off should be considered carefully from the different experts interested in this problem, such as physicians, sociologists, psychologists and others. At the end, probably nobody would shoulder the full responsibility. This could mean, in fact, to abandon guns or dynamite because they are considered dangerous to handle, and go back to bows and arrows, thus almost unarmed in front of certain serious, resistant and dangerous obesity.

While I am thinking about the conclusion of this long and important topic, I remember an old western film of Hollywood. Three people were travelling on horseback: a beautiful woman, a wealthy businessman and a shady character, elegant and quick with his gun. The three are attacked by Indians and they escape only thanks to the ability with guns of the shady character. They manage thus to ford the river safe and sound. The film gives us the opportunity to make an amusing comparison with what we have discussed in this chapter. Well, the businessman and the woman should as soon as possible try to do their best to split their own ways from the gunman, after having thanked him. At all costs they have to clear off, and eventually run away relying on their own strength. In fact, if his intervention has been useful to save a delicate moment of their journey, trying to look for his support little by little would mean to put themselves in his hands (see the danger from the continuous and perennial use of anorectics).

---

4   By starting with administration of a third or half tablet, the percentage of intolerant subjects diminishes to 5 or even 3% (personal case histories).

The use of the hormone chorionic gonadotropin (HCG) in the obesity treatment

The use of this placentar hormone as slimming drug was widespread in Italy in the 70's and 80's. It is necessary to clarify that the attention from the experts on this issue was drawn by an English physician, a Mr. Simeons in 1954. Through an announcement to the authoritative review "Lancet", he formulated the hypothesis that the administration of this substance in small daily doses, combined with a very low calorie diet (500 a day), aided the disposal of abnormal fat deposit of our organism, as in the case of pregnant Indian women. In addition, the use of this drug (used in many other fields of medicine but for other reasons[1]) seemed it protected patients against all those ailments frequently occurring when you follow very drastic diets. Of course, the first experience everybody hastened to do, was to verify if the final result, following the diet but not injecting the hormone, was the same after 40 days of treatment.

Different researchers selected two groups of patients: the first followed the 500 calorie diet and injected daily the hormone; the second followed the same diet but with no injection.

The result was that between the group who injected the hormone and the other one who had only followed the diet, there was no substantial difference, either as to the loss of weight (at the end of the 40 days) or as to the characteristic ailments from drastic slimming treatment, that is weakness, giddiness, indisposition and so on.

These disadvantages, in fact, in the case histories of different authors who tried method by Simeons for a long time, occurred exactly in the same percentages, even if the patients had been injected or not.

In the very few cases I tried this system myself, it happened that these disadvantages occurred more in patients that were injected than in others who did not want to inject the hormone belonging to the same family and

---

[1] The main fields where this hormone is commonly used are: regular miscarriage, sterility, insufficient development of sexual organs.

following the 500 calorie diet. They even kept fit better[2]. It is pretty sure that in the inner sheet of the box, the pharmaceutical industries producing the drug have never believed or think advisable to include, among the others, the indication for obesity.

---

2   It is necessary to highlight that Simeons in a letter addressed to the management of the American Journal of Clinical Nutrition in 1963, he outlined that the main purpose of the injections of HCG was not to make people lose more weight in respect to those who did not inject it, but to promote the disposal of abnormal fat deposits.

The unnecessary use
(and potentially detrimental)
of diuretics to lose weight.

A group of drugs, which I condemn totally, if they are used to lose weight, are diuretics. I have seen many patients, using them before for reasons of force majeure, to put on even 3 kg in 48 hours only which were lost in the previous checkup.

What stupefies more is the peremptory statement that they have not, in the meantime, drunk huge quantity of liquid or however more than their usual habits.

Nobody has ever lost weight in the long run by using diuretics. When I meet patients for the first time and they declare to have used them for this reason until that moment continuously, I warn them about the success of the treatment.

Very often herbal tablets, apparently harmless, are very diuretic and laxative. They are proposed as elixir of health, only because you can buy them in herbalist's shop than at the chemist's.

The recurrent use of herbs: a way to detoxifying rather than losing weight.

Many people think that fasting (almost completely) for some days, while having in the meantime some detoxifying potions (even if under clinical observation), can be a good idea to regain a good form. This is a questionable and not enough tested assertion! Moreover, if they even hope to lose 10,15 or also 20 kilos by following this sort of method, this is the result of bad information and ignorance.

If you use these potions too often or in an excessive way, you can suffer, in the long run from intestine disorders, colitis and dehydration.

Fortunately this kind of treatment does not end with any uneasiness or noteworthy episodes for two reasons.

The first is that this kind of treatment is used by "the snobs of slimming treatment", those who try to lose simply 2 or 3 kilos overweight all their life, without success[1].

The second one is that these so-called patients, in the evening, are starving and feel worn out. As a consequence the book up a table at a trattoria and pig themselves with their friends.

A reassuring advance information for the readers: the Progressive Method does not imply any use of drugs.

The reason is the dietetic succession which is the basis of the Progressive Method.

Its balanced stages hardly ever provoke excess of appetite or slowdown in weight loss which requires acceleration of metabolism.

---

1   From the stories and reports of my patients, it emerges that they attended Beauty Farms mainly to meet some friends, have a look round and show up rather than for a real interest in losing weight. Pardon me, on the other hand, how many kilos could be lost in seven days?

The delusive use of computer in slimming diets.
It does not help you to find an alternative

First of all, we have to say that the use of the computer to lose weight is delusive.

From one side, the user relies on it to obtain a sort of mysterious and secret recipe.

From the other one, most of the patients who tried to use the computer before contacting me, at the beginning they felt surprised, later on they got tired of talking with a Robot. I will explain the reason.

If you used a computer, for instance, to get accurate mathematical answers, in this case, it would be almost agreeable to play with it.

But in the food field, and particularly in slimming diets, saying is one thing, and doing another. In fact, we have to consider wealth of feelings, former sufferings, hopes and frustrations, which cannot be reduced to sheer questions to ask a computer. It has been educated by the man and imitates the human behavior.

Moreover it must be pointed out that, before that the computer processes its diet, we must answer about hundred questions. Even the most well-disposed patients lose their temper in front of strange, poorly pertinent questions that try to emphasize, I wonder which hidden aspects of obeses personality. Probably, they simply want to attach importance to it.

Finally, here we have this longed-for diet: unexceptionable as to calorie counting, but often with a bad fault. The computer, which has been taught by men, cannot propose alternative ways to lose weight if they were not present in the mind of the programmer.

In addition, some computers I saw many years ago proposed foods in bizarre and eccentric times, just think of eating string beans with olive oil at 9 a.m. or vegetable soup four times a day.

In any case, I think that today we can find computers which have corrected this sort of problems.

SECOND PART

OBESITY TODAY

What are
the most important clinical
news for a subject?

After your name, family name and age, you should also declare your educational degree. It is a precious piece of information, since it highlights a person's level of maturity and education; that allows a health operator to understand what the real health conditions of patients are as well as their psyche by what they tell about themselves, their illnesses, their past slimming diets, their unresolved emotional problems, if any.

Being married and having children are other very important factors, especially as far as women are concerned; actually, they are not only indicative of the degree of physical stress a female organism suffers on the occasion of pregnancies, but also inform about their living standard which usually affects their diet.

For instance, a working woman often does not have much time to cook, and therefore her diet will not generally include all those dishes that, although not complicated, yet require a certain degree of domestic relax. The same applies to businessmen or simply to people who often eat in places other than their own home: it should be possible to have salt-free boiled courgettes or an onion soup and the like in restaurants. If, however, patients need also that kind of food, it is possible, when they are not at home, to make them follow their diet plan including classic restaurant dishes (pasta, roasted meat, etc.).

You should also take into account all the diseases and surgical interventions an organism has undergone throughout its life.

Some past diseases require a particular care. For instance, if you have been affected by contagious diseases or tuberculosis, typhus, blood rheumatism and generally long pathologies which, although overcome, have anyhow recently required all your physical energies (even if you are in convalescence). In medicine some diseases are often underestimated, whereas many minor pathologies are given more relevance than they deserve.

As far as pregnant women are concerned (as well as breast-feeding women), generally they ought to abstain from any slimming diet; the same applies to children, especially those under the age of 10 years old, although in case of fast or early developing juvenile obesity, it would be excellent to adopt a 2000 calorie health diet whereby you can start to reasonably control your children diet without depriving a fully developing young organism of anything.

The Progressive Method is an assured slimming system that can be followed without any problem by all those people who need it and whose general physical conditions are good.

The cycles envisaged for a wide range of cases bring, besides a loss of weight, many other benefits among which the most significant is a drop in the cholesterol rate, triglycerides, arterial hypertension values, glycaemia and insulin-resistance. The same applies to those who are not obese, and yet considerably overweight.

The reduction of adiposity, especially as far as men are concerned, concentrates mainly in the subcutaneous adipose panniculus of the abdomen, which today is considered as the main unfavourable index predictive of future serious pathologies such as diabetes, hyperuricemia, hypertriglycerimia, hypercholesteremia and cardiovascular damage.

Women's loss of weight mostly affects hips, abdomen and the upper part of thighs which remain muscular and firm. That is possible because in all diets contained in this book (even those at low calories!) the carbohydrate and protein rate, besides the entire list of mineral salts and vitamin factors, remain constantly well represented.

Furthermore it is important to highlight how the diets foreseen by my Method, without making use of drugs, relieve and often cure non complicated hepatic steatosis peculiar to people who eat and drink a lot (namely an increase in liver fat without viral infections), frequently bringing the normalization of the main direct and indirect indexes of hepatic functionality. In many cases (and I refer to all subjects), notwithstanding they are hypocaloric diets, we have sometimes noticed also a rise in red cells (and in sideremia!).

Learn to "feed yourself"
instead of
only "eating"

Since ancient times men have always desired and tried to have an harmonious figure: its achievement brought also favourable balances in the whole organism which, in short, might be translated in the Latin saying *"mens sana in corpore sano"*. Romans, for instance, paid great attention to their body, dedicating themselves to thermal activities during which the body, as everybody knows, has the opportunity to get rid of some of the poisons and toxins accumulated during periods of heavy diets. Nobody can deny that nowadays, owing to a chaotic and unbalanced diet, liver is one of the most stressed organs. It is a gland-laboratory where almost all the main chemical reactions leading to the neutralization of endogenous and exogenous toxins take place. Nature has given this important organ the hard daily task of turning all the injurious chemical substances, yet present in our diet (preservatives, etc.), into not dangerous products. Besides that, it deals with the inactivation of other poisons that are inhaled every day, among which unfortunately the carbon oxide emitted by car exhaust pipes ranks the first (one day we might be obliged to walk in downtown wearing gas masks).

Well, as if all that were not enough, we can do nothing better but adding to the poor quality of our diet and the unfavourable surrounding environment a further and even greater deterioration factor, adopting a wrong, fat diet which may cause hypercholesteremia and early arteriosclerosis.

Even though this does not mean that everybody will become obese, yet this kind of diet can easily cause an increase in liver fat (steatosis) which hinders the liver functioning and may cause the future onset of metabolism degenerative diseases such as arteriosclerosis, hyperlipidemia, heart attack, etc.

Of course, all people who follow this diet do not necessarily contract those illnesses; it is true, however, that you can apparently eat wonderfully, but actually feed on very bad things[1].

---

1   It seems that the caveman, paradoxically and with the proper comparison, had a better diet than ours (Thierry Souccard, Régime prehistorique, Science et avenir, may 2001).

35

Astronauts remain in space for many days, sometimes even for months: they are given scientific tasks whose accomplishment requires very fit bodies. Of course, in space shuttles you do not have any kitchen where to cook hot stews or delicious cakes (I think!). You can feed well by simply swallowing pills (or ready frozen meals, sorry but I. am not expert of space medicine), and on the contrary you can feed badly by gulping down the most tasty of our dishes. I have carried my speech too far, but there are many other ways of following good sense, which is always in between.

If we carried out opinion polls, asking people which disease is the cause of the highest number of deaths all over the world, I am sure the majority would consider cancer as the most responsible disease. On the contrary, very few. people would indicate arteriosclerosis, cardiovascular diseases and arterial hypertension as the real and main cause, even though they are unfortunately first on the list of the world causes of death.

What are the aims
to reach
for a correct
diet

In Italy there are at last less deaths from heart attack. In March 1983, the 20% of Italians has gone out from the "high-risk" zone. The reason is that they have started following a diet where they have applied some dietetic principles "without bordering on the ghost of hunger". The diet consists in the use of cereals, rice and pulses to employ long-chemical-chain starches and natural carbohydrates. In addition, there is less castor sugar which should be responsible for the tendency towards diabetes and other serious pathology (arteriosclerosis, and so on).

Salt must not exceed more than two or three grams a day. Such recommendations coincide with those expressed by the United States Senate Select Committee[1].

Even the Ministry of Health hand the Italian government have started for some years to speak about a revaluation of the Mediterranean diet. That is, a diet with less animal fats and more olive oil, less meat and more food. Sugars are not inferior to 60% and must be natural, that is, taken from milk, fruit, cereals, pulses, potatoes. You should try to leave out more and more refined sugar and use the raw one[2].

What strikes more is that the Americans declared that Mediterranean diet was, after all, one of the best in the world. Just think we followed it every day and we had never noticed it! We are always the usual absent-minded!

Let us speak in details about the food objectives to reach according to the outcome of the United State Committee. They are important because they have a didactic function as to the normal diet of a sound subject. From the other side, this offers interesting hints as to the wrong diet of obeses which is identical to the hypercaloric one of western peoples. We hope that, in the

---

1   United States Senate Select Committee on Nutrition and Human Needs.
2   These concepts have always been the primary objective of my consulting room. At the beginning I risked to be look askance at, and with suspect when I prescribed rice, pasta, potatoes, starchy food and raw honey. Some of them even asked me if by chance they had mistaken the address!

future, this diet will modify and coincide with the food rules by the United States Senate Committee.

The problem in this country is very urgent because the total consumption of fats was the 42% some years ago. It is a long way to reduce it to the foreseen 30%. The whole American situation comprehended years ago the following data: carbohydrates 46% (24% formed of sugars and 22% of starches), fats 42%, proteins 12%. The targets for the future, concerning the different countries, show the following data: carbohydrates 58% (15% of sugars and 43% of starches), fats 30%, proteins, 12%.

In few words, the 12% of fats less should favor sugars on their whole. Inside them, however, in turn, about a 10% must shift toward the raw ones, that is in favor of starches and long chemical chain polysaccharides[3].

Therefore, less fats, more bread, more pasta, more pulses and less sweets.

The Italian situation is better than the American one since the fat consumption, in our country, is roundabout 33%. Therefore almost 10% less.

In the Italian diet, food fats are divided into: polyunsaturated 6%, monounsaturated 14% and saturated 13%, while in the recommended diet they will modify into 10% polyunsaturated, 10% monounsaturated and 10% saturated.

The dietetic goals have been adopted by the National Committee on Nutrition which includes seven major medical associations in the United States for the study of food, nutrition and dietetics (Select Committee on Nutrition and Human Needs, US Senate: Dietary Goals for the United States, Washington D. C., Govt., Prtg. Pff. Dec. 1977).

Energy balance. Eat daily as many calories as your organism needs. If you are obese, or even simply excess weight, lower the intake of daily calories. We remind you, in fact that the insurance companies consider in their tables the weight when they issue life insurances. Obese people, statistically speaking, are at high-risk as to coronary disease.

Carbohydrates and sugar. The total consumption of sugars must form about the 58% of total daily calories. The ideal partition states that the 48% must be formed by complex carbohydrates (starches, polysaccharides). Only the 10% of the total calories can be represented by refined sugars contained in syrups, jams, sweets.

---

3   *The last recommended portions, in order of time carried out by technical bodies in charge, would recommend in all countries to raise the share of carbohydrates at about the 63%, proteins 10-11%, fats 26-27%.*

A diet rich in starches ensures in addition an adequate contribution of fibers, useful to reduce several pathological processes of the colon, and to improve the glucose tolerance in diabetes.

Proteins. Limiting the protein consumption at about 12-15%. Try to reduce the proteins of animal origin (meat, fish, eggs, cheese, milk) in favor of proteins of vegetable origin.

(Unfortunately such food recommendations, as to daily proteins, are not applicable to a slimming diet, because the sources of vegetable proteins have always a high content of starches which increase the number of calories (lentils, rice, beans, chickpeas, broad beans, bread, pasta, fruit). Notwithstanding this highly restricting factor, that is the high caloric content of starchy food, my consulting room can claim the credit for having always, since the beginning of my professional activity in the early 70's, preferred starchy food when I was drawing up low-calorie slimming diets (even the lowest). These concepts were evident to me and the United States Senate Committee later confirmed them in a sensational way.

Cholesterol. Reducing the consumption of cholesterol to about 300 mg a day. This is a prescription which is not always easy to follow since cholesterol is contained in a lot of food. In eggs (a single egg contains 200 mg), butter, custard, fat cheese, fat meat, offal, some fat fish. The relative difficulty in modifying a level of concentration in blood through its reduction in the diet is due to the fact that, with a minor contribution, the organism reacts by synthesizing it, that is by producing it. Its normalization in the diet is part of a precise project from CNR.

Sodium. Limiting the administration of sodium by reducing the consumption of salt to no more than 3 grams a day.

There is no doubt by now that the results of studies made by different scientists have reached the conclusion that the elevated consumption of common salt (that is sodium chloride) provokes arterial hypertension in predisposed subjects.

Since the number of these subjects is huge, practically, if you could make sure that the consumption of salt is low for everybody, and for our entire life, that would be a great success. In fact, the most devastating social scourge, which takes a heavier toll of lives than cancer, would be curable in most cases, by adopting the most stupid of remedies.

I would be really interested, beyond the polemical humor, in knowing the reasons which prevent from the uncontrollable rise in the price of salt, so that it would not certainly be eaten anymore with such a similar abuse.

Fats. Reducing the consumption of total fats to about 30% of the total calories. In America this reduction must practically last a long time, since the actual consumption is about 43%. Luckily, in Italy, the target is more attainable, since our consumption must be reduced of only 3 percentage points, that is from 33% to 30% of the total calories. It is useful however to remember, even if this is a technical aspect, that this ideal 30% must be divided into 10% each for saturated fats, or rather coming from nearly animal origin, 10% from monounsaturated fats, 10% from polyunsaturated fats of vegetables origin (olive oil and so on). Reduce saturated fat consumption to account for about 10% of total calorie intake.

THIRD PART

LOSE WEIGHT EASILY
AND GET RID
OF DIET ADDICTION

What should be
by far
the best
slimming diet

It is very simple; by now I think that many should already recognize it, even if roughly, by using the fundamental scheme.

FUNDAMENTAL SCHEME	
NUMBER → OF KILOS ← LOST	1. Length of the treatment 2. Entity of sacrifice 3. Possible use of drugs 4. Respect of the general health conditions 5. Steadiness of the result obtained 6. Quantity and quality of clinical check-ups 7. Degree of the doctor's professionality 8. Global cost of the fee.
Good quality of a slimming treatment = the optimal relationship between number of kiloslost, from one side, and all the other factor, from the other one.	

The best treatment should assure the loss of a considerable number of kilos in a nor very short neither too long period of time (not more than 2-3 months at the most), without too heavy sacrifices, making a limited use or, better, not use at all of drugs, under the control of a doctor specialized in Dietetics and Food Science.

During the treatment patients are to undergo serious clinical controls, regularly checking not only their weight and blood pressure, but also their general state of health before continuing their diet. The best diet should, therefore, annul the tendency to fatness in patients for good so that they might go back to a normal daily diet without running the risk of putting on weight again.

All that might seem very easy to do in theory. In practice, however, it is quite difficult if you do not have an expert guide and all these favourable conditions do not occur at the same time. It is like winning at the National Lottery: guessing 3,4 numbers is not enough to be among the winners. This example is really pertinent.

Let us consider one by one and in detail some different cases that may occur during, a slimming diet.

After reading them, nobody can pretend to have doubts or have misunderstood.

I case. Only few kilos have been lost and yet all the other conditions have been respected: clearly the target has been missed.

II case. This time a certain number of kilos have been lost: in order to achieve this result, however, the treatment has implied almost an year of sacrifices: modest result.

III case. A good many kilos have been lost, but at the cost of fasts and very hard sacrifices: poor result (we all know that if we starve, we lose weight, there is no need of a dietician for that).

IV case. A good many kilos have been lost without giving up anything, but that has been possible thanks to anorectic drugs and amphetamines, which, administered since the very beginning and in strong doses, have managed to annul any kind of willpower, zeroing any appetite: very poor result. There is a 80-90% probability that in a very near future we will see a considerable rise in appetite (and in weight).

V case. A good many kilos have been lost, the treatment length has been optimum, the sacrifices really bearable, no drugs have been administered, no problem has been caused to the patient's health: very good. However, there can be another problem: the result is very long in stabilizing or does not stabilize at all. Therefore, the conclusion is that once again the target has been missed.

VI case. All the aforementioned conditions (this time there is no point in repeating them) have been respected: the treatment, however, has been very expensive: questionable result (even though the majority of the obese people do not pay great attention to the economic side of the matter, for they would pay any price to get rid of their condition).

What you can do
to get
as closer as possible
to the ideal diet

First of all, one should start making efforts since the very beginning, without losing time discussing how many kilos are to be lost. I remember a friend of mine who had to go by car from Naples to Milan: instead of leaving very early in the morning and driving along the roads and highways he knew quite well, before leaving he began to think about the possibilities of going along alternative roads, even if they were 800 or 1000 km far away.

Similarly, many people, who actually should lose no more than 15 kilos, waste their time talking about the fact that maybe they should lose 20 or even 30 kilos, as if the road that leads to the loss of 20 or 30 kilos did not pass through the loss of 15 kilos. The most common mistake is made, however, by people who decide to adopt a starvation diet since the very beginning in order to end the treatment within few days. All these people (and there are many of them, even among educated people) behave the same way as those who start going up the stairs by rushing and maybe climbing three steps at a time, without thinking they are to reach the IX-X floor. At first sight, the result will seem amazing, and they will be sure they have gained a huge advantage over those who, on the contrary, start going up at a steady pace.

After they have lost, by starvation diets and frustrating fasts, almost a kilo and a half in the first three days, they lose just a half kilo – a kilo in the following 3 days and 2 hectograms per day in the next 3 days, till the moment when, around the tenth day of diet, they stop losing weight even though – and that is terrible – they continue their starvation diet. At that point, the initial amazement and euphoria start being replaced by disappointment. All the people who had been informed that finally a miraculous slimming method had been found, yet are not informed about this discouraging latest piece of news; therefore they go on thinking and informing other people that finally someone has found a quick way of losing weight. Certainly, if the person who has decided to heroically undergo such a starvation diet were as honest as to inform everybody that it was a false alarm and that unfortunately reality is totally different, then this chain would be immediately interrupted.

45

Unfortunately, however, we can not expect everybody is ready to publicly acknowledge their mistakes: that is why some misunderstandings get more and more complicated as the time goes by, instead of becoming clear.

This kind of disappointment is frequent among people who follow drastic slimming methods, adopting since the very beginning very poor diet that remain so for the whole treatment period. Actually in these cases, after having immediately lost some kilos, then patients will remain steady at the same weight or even put on again some of the kilos lost in the very first days; every time they will check their weight on the scales, they will live a real nightmare, feeling even worse when after 30 days they see other people, who have started their diet in a much more relaxed way, as slimmer as they are. It is just as when in the highway, driving at 140 km/hour, we overtake another car going at 120 km/hour: as soon as we stop, however, after less than 3-4 minutes, we see that car, which should have taken twice as much as we would, passing by.

At that moment I guess many of you have thought: we have wasted much more petrol and run many more potential risks just to arrive few minutes before!

What we can do
to keep
in the long term
our results permanent

After many years spent studying obesity, I can confidently affirm that generally to the general average of my patients, once the period of dropping calories as well as the period of the calorie rise is over (which constitute all together the Progressive Method by Doctor D'Antoni, see page 56), it takes not more than 4 weeks to stabilize the result they have achieved[1] (see page 57).

After this length of time, subjects shall follow a free and as various as possible diet, without sacrifices and yet without excesses, according to the needs of their new weight[2].

Frequently, in order to foster a better balance of the diencephalon nerve centre (set-point), a steady and not competitive physical exercise has turned out to be very useful, provided that it does not trigger the mechanism of an uncontrolled consumption of food, which is unfortunately frequent among people who practice physical activities.

Certainly, as often happens in medicine, there are always easy cases (for example, some slimmer subjects, who, owing to circumstances beyond their own control, could not accurately follow the second phase which foresees the rise of calories, and yet do not have weight problems any more, even after many years, showing that they have stabilized the result by simply decreasing calories!).

Sometimes there are some more difficult situations where the definitive stabilization of weight is a bit more complicated. They are mostly subjects who have tried to lose weight tens of times (the so-called yo-yo syndrome). In these cases, a slower approach to the definitive number of calories to be assumed every day may help. I must admit, however, that in more than 20 years of professional activity I have never seen patients, who has carefully followed the

---

1   if we want to, we can consider this delicate period of adjustment as a real exercise for the patients who, even if in the long run, can always themselves guided and corrected in time, if necessary.

2   By following always the constant formula already mentioned on page 12, that is 30-35 cal. per Kg. of weight = daily total calories.

instructions and terms of the Progressive Method, achieving a good result, then having to follow long reduced diets in order to stabilize their weight.

Between these two ends - the first one represented by subjects who do not need to follow the second stage of calorie rise as the Method envisages, and the other one by patients who, on the contrary, in order to stabilize the result they have achieved, have to pay greater attention as soon as they come back to a normal diet (see note in the previous page) – there is the general average of subjects, who, besides maintaining the new weight by adopting the suggested definitive diet, are generally more refractory to put on weight again, even though the variety of cases may show differences from one another. My collaborators and I (we are a private firm) are anyhow sure that, since this kind of cases are really numerous, if we managed to carry out a real, more in-depth statistical survey (capable of prolonging the follow-up), we would have pleasant surprises!

Of course, this various record of cases includes also patients whose results can not be evaluated because they are neither part of the general average nor of the two minorities, for they are people who do not complete the whole cycle, interrupting it at various stages - during either the decrease of calories, or immediately after, or the new increase of them, or the first days of stabilization of the achieved results.

The risk of making our slimming diet chronic. Once you reach the end of the cycle, it is necessary to get rid of diet addiction

If the dangers of a lightning treatment are now well known (tiredness, drop in the arterial pressure, overall fatigue, nervous tension, loss of muscle tone, etc., and moreover without achieving best results than those given by more relaxed diets), maybe nobody has never analyzed the risks of slow and prolonged diets, since so far the other kind of treatment - namely the too quick one - has been regarded as the most dangerous.

Actually, the risks of slow treatments are as insidious and dangerous as those of the quick ones. Let us see now in detail how this kind of treatment works.

The diet given at the moment of the first examination (if there is a real check-up) usually remains as it is throughout the treatment or is replaced by another diet which has the same number of daily calories but envisages a different kind of dishes. This precaution is to be taken especially when the treatment is decided by personnel that is expert in this field but not medical, for this way a patient is definitely more unlikely to have health problems. If, on the one hand, this way of treating can protect (even though relatively) patients, on the other hand the treatment becomes too long and exhausting. Certainly, if you reduce the quantity of calories an organism takes in every day, then it immediately loses a few kilos.

The path we have ahead, however, is not so easy as the first steps we have done.

The most important factor allowing a further loss of kilos is the progressive reduction of food.

Without this measure - alas, painful, but necessary and irreplaceable - all the other moves we might make will not lead to appreciable results.

Therefore, people who follow a slimming diet envisaging the administration of the same number of calories for the whole treatment period run the risk of becoming chronic; that is to say that, even though they do not reduce their daily calories, they anyway eat less than other people without achieving their target[1], or achieving it at least after 1-2 years.

Furthermore, these subjects get so accustomed to eating less than they should that, if they start again to have a normal diet, they will put immediately on again the few kilos they have lost. We could compare them with those who, ignoring their doctor's advice, instead of following the treatment in the prescribed time, decide to follow it as they like. As a consequence of that, if they decide to interrupt the assumption of those particular pills, they will immediately fall ill again with just the disease they have been treating by assuming those pills, which have therefore become absolutely necessary for them.

---

1   It is necessary that a slimming cycle has a strategy. It is as a war films when generals gathered together take stock of the military situation, looking at the map of the area to be conquered and evaluating which means they can use: airplanes, tanks, infantry. I am sorry to speak about these aspects but they are the only ones which make the comparison clear. For example, one of this which gives exactly the idea is the general who, together with his tired troops, wants at any cost, to go on with his advance to conquer another strip of territory instead of stopping and acquiring strength (the equivalent is who wants to lose at any cost more weight and bring the kilos lost from 17 to 20, or from 12 to 15. It is very easy that the enemy (obesity) organizes a counteroffensive and takes back his territories.

FOURTH PART

ILLUSTRATION AND EXPLANATION OF THE PROGRESSIVE METHOD

The basis of the Progressive Method is the Mediterranean diet: how to lose many kilos without ever using drugs, keeping a normal appetite and a perfect shape.

The basic diet of the Progressive Method is the famous Mediterranean diet.

I stress the word "famous" because it seems it was newly discovered almost to create a novelty. Instead the truth is that everybody knew it and followed it. Even our ancestors, before the Greeks and Romans, with no class distinction, because it was the only one available, to live in good health without alternatives.

We are speaking of every day food, such as bread which has always been the basic food for the survival of the human race. Firstly rough loaves, today appetizing food baked by our bakery's. It is uncomprehensible how it is possible to get rid of bread in a human diet considering that probably we have already in our chromosomes the genes corresponding to its digestion.

Together with eggs, meat and milk we go back to the cave man, as well as with vegetables, fruit and so on. Even the sugar cane gave already, from time immemorial, its fruit. Firstly, it was precious like gold, then, with the advent of western wealth, it was despised and avoided "like a poison".

Thank goodness that recently this blessed "Mediterranean diet" is trendy.

But let me ask a question. Before this sort of "trend", how did we eat? Could you refresh my memory? Frankly, I do not remember something else (since ever!).

The homo erectus gets on well with the so-called Mediterranean diet because he was born and grown up for 50,000 years (according to others also until 200,000) with these food habits which foresee more than 50% of carbohydrates (between slow and fast).

How many generations would be necessary to develop a genetic heritage which would allow to do without, by adapting well to the condition of everlasting acetonomial?

The problem is that along with the traditional way of eating new habits overlapped. This has been caused by the spread of wealth. If we have a generous main course, we add a second course which is equally seasoned and generous. Normally we eat the sweet too and snacks increase from meal to meal.

Therefore, pasta or rice is not responsible for putting on weight, rather sauces, sweets as constant habit, walnuts, hazelnuts, dates and so on.

Here is a list of some savory vegetable sauces for pasta, tagliatelle or rice:

- eggplants, tomato, garlic, basil;
- zucchinis, garlic, parsley;
- eggplants, tomato, onions and parsley;
- cauliflower, onions;
- artichokes, garlic, parsley.

Why the Progressive Method does not need drugs.

The answer is simple: the stages of the dietetic ups and downs represent metabolic moments which are particularly suitable for the needs of our organism. Therefore, the well organized caloric succession in the different diets (dietetic ups and downs) always allows a well balanced supply which protects the patients' appetite from all those feelings of unsatisfaction and disorder provoking the interruption of the diet.

Soon after the review from the whole press, different enthusiastic confirmations from readers followed. We received uncountable personal proofs, many from obese physicians, which state the great success of method which they applied to themselves and their patients.

The theory the Progressive Method by Dr. D'Antoni is based on

Progressive Method means that, once you begin this slimming cycle, it is necessary to use other diets in a very precise progression, if you want to keep on losing weight. These slimming programs have to be different depending on the stage, which is related to the weight already lost and that one you have still to lose to reach your ideal weight.

This is why the Method comprehends seven mains situations of obesity and six fundamental progressive caloric levels: the first at 2000 calories, the second at 1600, the third at 1400, the fourth at 1200, the fifth at 900, the sixth 600[1]. During the passages it is possible to lose, with some differences according to the circumstances, about 15 kg in 50 - 60 days. When you reach the most low diet, you start to rise the various caloric levels already went through during the drop: from 600 to 900, 1200, 1400, 1600 and 2000.

During the rise, normally, you still lose a couple of kilos. This happens, even if you increase the calories introduced daily in a progressive way.

When you come back to the initial starting level (to the diets of 1400 - 1600 - 2000 calories), the aim is to return, always gradually, to your normal everyday diet.

You can obtain this by defining the <u>definitive counting of your calories according to the formula already mentioned several times</u>: 30-35 cal x kg of bodily weight = necessary daily energy.

---

1   In this case we consider the dietetic itinerary of subject called "B" (see page *65)* who begins from 1600 calories. This is one of the commonest situations that is a man weighing 90 kg instead of 75 (ideal weight). The subjects called A1 and A2 (respectively a man weighing 80 kg instead of 65 and a woman weighing 70 kg instead of 55) have to start both with a 1400 calorie diet and should lower their intake to 600 calories, even if for some days, so that they complete the caloric ups and downs and bewilder the set-point (see following chapter). Vice versa very obese patients (subjects C – C1) will have to start the first of the two cycles from 2000 calories (see page 67) and consider as last caloric level of this first cycle that of 700 calories, reaching in this way a weight of about 90 kg. Successively, after a recommended interval of about some months they will follow a second cycle. For convenience and simplicity, this has been identified with that of the subject B. <u>Important warning</u>: all the suggested cycles can be repeated at least after 3-4 months from the last new rise of calories.

<u>Let us give some examples:</u>

Subject A_1: weight obtained at the end of Progressive Method (starting from 80 kg) = kg 65x35 cal/kg (man) = 2300 (about) daily calories allowed;

Subject A_A: weight obtained at the end of the cycle = kg 65x30 cal/kg (woman) = 1800 daily calories allowed (always moderate physical activity);

Subject B: weight obtained at the end of the cycle = kg 75x35 cal/kg weight (man) = 2500 daily calories allowed (moderate physical activity);

Subject B_1: weight obtained at the end of the cycle = kg 75x30 = about 2200 (woman – suggested not more than 1800 - 2000 calories / day);

Subject C: (a period of some months between first and second cycle during which the weight is still 90 kg) kg 90x32 cal/kg = 2800 daily calories (man);

Subject C_1: kg 90x30-26 cal/kg = 2300 daily calories (woman)[2].

<u>The difference between the calories reached</u> by the six subjects at the end of the respective rises <u>and the final ones they are allowed to</u>, must be also added to the daily diet <u>according a recommended rhythm of about 300 - 400 calories a week</u>. They can postpone eventually this addition if they notice a tendency to put on weight.

<u>In this book, the subject of dietetics has been dealt with in a scientific way but popular too. I have even listed the analytical composition of food (logical analysis) which, for the first time, is offered to the wide readers' public.</u> Well, by consulting these tables, readers could also choose by themselves the food containing the necessary calories to make the diet increase of 300 – 400 calories. There are many other factors to keep in mind: one of these is that, for example, you could choose food which could upset the optimal percentages because they contain many carbohydrates, lipids or proteins.

It is therefore better you use, for this reason, the diets already included and elaborated. For example, for this purpose, the subject A_2 could easily use the 1600 calorie diet (page 65) as an intermediate stage to get from 1400 to 1800 (final diet). The same concept can be valid also for subject A_1: from 1400 → 1600 → 2000 (Health Diet, page119). The subjects B and C will add, to those of 2000, some other food to fill the last stage until 2600 calories.

---

2   This is the period in which the weight starting from 105 arrives to 90 kg (between first and second cycle). Successively after 3-4 months she will begin her second cycle starting from the 1600 calories diet. Practically subjects C – C1 as their second cycle run over again the same itinerary of subjects B – B1. This has been made to simplify enormously the Method.

Since this last diet is very energetic, if you add 500 calories according to your own taste, this is not a problem. Except if you do not think to burn 500 calories using 70 gr. of butter or 100 gr. of sugar or 300 gr. of meat with many fats!).

Pay attention: I seize the opportunity to say that for the readers of some countries (included USA) it is necessary to use roast-beef[3], since in some charts of food composition, beef is meant to contain 20 gr. of fats for hundred grams (USA). In Italy, only very fat beef, or even pork, contain this percentage of lipids, making calories raise from 100-120 (roast-beef) to 380 - 400 for only hundred grams! Of course, you should not be on diet for the rest of your life, following the calculations made in this book. The target I want to reach with the readers is to make them grow an individual conscience by offering a correct way of eating, nourishing and scientific, which does not involve any sacrifice. The majority of subjects, in the long term, (at least those who have lost weight with this book in Italy) have told to have got used, almost automatically, during their diets, to plan the amount of calories allowed, being able to choose different appetizing food.

This slimming program, I created and nicknamed Progressive Method, was born from the necessity to find a strategic winning choice against obesity.

The difference between my method and any other traditional system, which always foresees the carrying out of constant diets, is the following as to calories:

Say the subject of the first example (case A_1), after having reached 76 kg from 80 during the first 20 days of the cure, should decide to carry on always with the about 1200 calorie diets.

In this case, if he would not follow the diets of 900 and 600 calories, after having lost the first 4 kg in 20 days, he would not lose easily the following kilos.

In conclusion, the result after 60 days would be, at best, about the half (or less) than that he would have reached with the Progressive Method. Even if theoretical preambles[4] would take for granted a result (at the end of 60 days) of about 12 or 13 kg, by using a diet of 1200 calories for a patient weighing 80 kg, practically this does not take place because of so far unknown mechanisms. The main problem seems to be the fact that the diencephalic nerve center *(set-point)* defends the previous weight strenuously and tenaciously.

Only by reducing the number of calories progressively, the diencephalic nerve center is unblocked, disorientated, and allows at last the loss of excess

---

3　　You can also use some other white meat as specified in the different diets.

4　　That is foreseeing the loss of 1 kg every 6000 calories missing (or according to others, every 7000).

kilos[5]. However, pay attention to respect the instructions until the end. If not, you could have some surprises during the rise of calories, with unexpected rebounds of weight; it would be as an alarm signal which, not having been neutralized successfully, can compromise a result which seemed already acquired.

---

5   When the degree of knowledge about the functioning of set-point will improve with new acquisitions, we will be able to single out the reasons of hormonal or biochemical nature which allow the Progressive Method to defeat obesity easily and to cause a basic refractoriness at the end of the treatment, according to the cases. Seen the present tendency in all living beings to create situation of stable balance, a first explanation could already be the continuous variation of calories in the Progressive Method, which would provoke therefore a real bewilderment of the set-point, during which the general action of check it exercises over the metabolism of obese people would be neutralized (Theory of Set-Point Shock by Dr. Michele D'Antoni,

The dietetic ups and downs
foreseen for the different subjects

Among all the possible forms of obesity, we have thought it right to propose seven examples which reflect with the evidence the most frequent practical cases. We have respectively gathered them into three groups: "A", "B" and "C". Each group contains different subjects: → group A contains subjects A_1 -A_A - A_2; group B contains: B - B_1; group C contains: C – C_1.

The subjects present in group A are of either sex, with different weights and a common dietetic path from 1400 to 600 calories and vice versa.

The group "B" (B – B_1) still supposes only people with an excess weight of 14 - 15 kg. The group "C" includes real obese patients with more than 30 kg in excess (C – C_1 man/woman).

Readers must base themselves, as far as possible, on the example closer to their situation. Much more severe obesity has not been taken into consideration and therefore illustrated, because such heavy problems require absolutely a constant specialist medical check-up. The same applies for all those particular pathologies that even if they do not represent serious medical conditions, cannot be treated without the continuous contact between physician and patient, by personalizing the treatment case by case (that is not absolutely the aim of this book).

First group - Subject A_1

Man, height: about 1.67 m. Weight: 80 kg. Frame: medium. Job: sedentary.

The estimated calories he intakes are 3200 a day. Calories necessary to keep the same weight (which is excessive) of 80 kg are about 2800. If this subject would succeed in reaching the ideal weight of 64-65 kg the calories necessary to keep this weight stable would be 2300 (about) a day.

First group - Subject A_A

Woman, height: 1.70 m. Weight: 80 kg. Frame: medium. Job: light.

The estimated calories she intakes are at least 2800 a day.

Calories necessary to keep the same weight (which is excessive) of 80 kg are about 2800. Ideal weight: about 64-65 kg. In this case, it would be necessary about 30 cal x body weight kg = 1800 daily calories.

Drop of calories of subjects A₁ - A_A (A₁ is a man - A_A is a woman)

To lose weight from 80 to 70 kg in 50 days same (diet for the two subjects):

Weight reached (starting from 80 kg)	Number of kilos lost	Number of dropping days of (on average)	Calories of the diet
78	2	10	1400
76	2	10	1200
73-72	3-4	20	900
70	2	10	600
70	10	50	--------------------

The above-mentioned subjects lose 4 kg in the first 20 days, by following diets of 1400 and 1200 calories. Afterwards, 3 kg more in the following 20 days, by following a diet of 900 calories. Finally, 2 kg more if they go down to 600 calories. They can lose even 10 kg in 50 days (only in the dropping stage of calories).

Rising of calories for subjects A₁ - A_A after the first 50 days of diet

Weight reached at the end of 50 days = 70 kg

Weight reached (starting from 70 kg)	Numbers of kilos further lost	Number of days of rising	Progressive calories of the rising diet
69/68	1-2	10	from 600 to 900
68/67	1-0	10	from 900 to 1200
67/66	1-0	10	from 1200 to 1400
67/66	2-3	30	--------------------

The subjects, during the rising of calories (from 600 to 1400), not only do not put on weight but on the contrary they lose 2/3 kg more (as normal situation). In some cases the kilos lost for both man and woman are different. The woman, considered the same initial weight and calories, is slightly disadvantaged as to the man. The rule is however not compulsory. On the contrary it may happen the contrary (which is not so rare).

As to the diets of 600 and 900 calories, I would like to be more precise about the fact that these diets can ensure enough vitamins and minerals supplied by 700 g of vegetables and fruit a day. However, from one side, for an excess of precaution which characterizes each page of this book, I would be tempted to advise you to ask your physician to prescribe some integrators containing further vitamins and mineral salts. On the other one, considered that the values achieved by these diets are far more than sufficient (as you can see by consulting the related charts) I do not see the point in giving you this piece of, advice[1].

These diets frequently contain already some big "pills" of natural vitamins with a rotation mechanisms. For example, 1 day the egg out of four days other menus which do not contain it. Eggs are rich in some of the most vitamins and minerals. On the contrary, if you eat them hard boiled (better if you keep them in the fridge, like fresh fruit), they remove the feeling of hunger from your stomach. Of course, we do not have to ignore the problem of cholesterol contained in the yolk (about 200 mg an egg)[2].

Remember, however, that a plain hen's egg , in its simplicity and low content of calories (only 76!) can offer you first of all a good feeling of satiety because if it is hard boiled, the gastric juices need almost 3 hours to digest it. Moreover, it contains noble proteins, iron (6 mg), calcium (150 mg), potassium, vitamin A (640 nanograms of equivalent retinol), vitamin K, zinc, vitamin B12, as well as plenty of Piridossina, Biodina, Tiamina. And do not forget that an egg, everywhere in the world, costs only few cents. It is true that its use has been always neglected especially in slimming diets[3].

Warning: diabetics and hypertensives must reduce, during the diets of 900 and 600 calories, the daily dosage of their drugs, since (and this is one of the positive aspects of this method) in a different way from subject to subject, we can observe a restoration of the organism's compromised functions (in this case the lowering of glycemia and bloody pressure).

---

1   Maybe some particular attention should be paid by the readers living in very industrialized countries (USA at the top) where the abundant use of frozen food do provoke a drop of vitamins in vegetables and fruit.

2   The worldwide maximum amount of cholesterol we can intake from food on a conservative level is 300 mg a day. Since the content in yolks is about 200 mg, the average subject hardly introduces in the same day, food containing more than 100 mg (for example, more than 150 gr. of meat, cheese or fish). It is necessary to remember that however our organism produces by itself cholesterol when necessary.

3   However, I want to reassure at once all of you, by telling you that, even in those days containing the egg, the cholesterol does not exceed the recommended or allowed one (that is 300 mg a day). I think it is very frustrating eating only the white (as it is recently recommended in last books or magazines) and throw away the precious yolk in the bin or give it to your pets. This how neurosis starts!

Let's go on with the illustration of the rising and dropping of calories related to the commonest situations of obesity.

First group - Subject A$_2$

Woman, height: 1.62 m. Actual weight: 70 kg. Ideal weight: 55-56 kg. Frame: medium-light. Job: light (housewife, employee). The estimated calories she intakes are 2800 a day. Calories necessary to keep the ideal weight of 55-56 kg: 1800 (32 cal x 55-56 = 1800 daily calories.

Drop of calories of subjects A$_2$ to lose weight from 70 to 61 kg in 48 days

Weight reached (starting from 70 kg)	Number of kilos lost	Number of dropping days (on average)	Calories of the diet
68	2	10	1400
66	2	10	1200
63/64	3/4	20	900
62/61	1/2	8	600
61	9-10	48	----------------------

The above-mentioned subject loses 4 kg in the first 20 days, by following diets of 1400 and 1200 calories. Afterwards, 3 kg more in the following 20 days, by following a diet of 900 calories. Finally, 2 kg more if she goes down to 600 calories. On average she can lose 9/10 kg in 48 days during the only dropping stage of calories.

Rising of calories for subject A$_2$ after the first 48 days of diet

Weight reached at the end of 48 days = 61 kg

Weight reached (starting from 61 kg)	Numbers of kilos further lost	Number of days of rising	Progressive calories of the rising diet
59/60	2/1	10	from 600 to 900
58/59	1/0	10	from 900 to 1200
57/58	1/0	10	from 1200 to 1400
57/58	2/3	30	

The subject, during the rising of calories (from 600 to 1400) in about 30 days, not only does not put on weight but on the contrary she loses 2/3 kg more (as normal situation). In some cases the total kilos lost in 78 days (48 days of dropping of calories and 30 days of rising) can also be more than those included in the scheme. However, this is always an average of results obtained by different subjects. We have also to consider the variables.

I make a pause, before continuing the analysis of the charts, to say that the results given so far and the next ones, cannot bind the Author and the Publisher, even if they come from the general average and a wide experience and experimentation. They cannot guarantee that anybody, among the readers, even if they can identify themselves in one of the subjects described in the examples, can mathematically get the result described in the charts. The main reasons are the following:

1. If the subjects transgress the diet and to which extent (they are the only ones to know it) or if they already intake much less calories than those foreseen.

2. If the subject has tried countless times to lose weight (the so-called yo-yo syndrome). This means weight loss of a couple of kilos followed by weight regain. In these cases, as everybody knows, the metabolism of this kind of patient is more used to cyclical restrictions and the set-point will do its best to make the introduced calories be enough until the end. That is why, in order to bewilder it, to follow the 600 calorie diets. Today these sort of diets are considered safe, especially if they are well balanced and with a good protein minimum level[4].

3. The age of subjects, their habits, case histories, social classes and so on. If the patient is a woman, it is of great importance if she is on the pill, if she had children, aborts, if she follows a hormone therapy or takes cortisone. For people of either sex, it is important if they can cook at home or are obliged to eat in a fast-food, where sauces play the lord and master. However, long live optimism! Very often I meet people for the first time who are disheartened because they have tried 10-20 times and they have lost few kilos in a bad way. Well then, the kilos lost are often more than those described in the charts!! Other times, on the contrary, I met patients who kept on repeating that they only needed to go on a diet to lose the overweight kilos. Goodness

---

4   These caloric levels are often used in University Centers and Italian hospitals against obesity-resistant. We had used them since the beginning of 80s, even on subjects working in stressful conditions, such as pilots, captains and so on. We have had no problems of any kind, if they were elaborated with a good experienced eye.

me! How difficult it was to make them reach their goal! On the other hand, there was no need to see a dietician, if their situation was exactly how they had told us.

Second group - Subject B

Man, height: 1.80 m. Frame: medium. Job: sedentary. Initial weight: 90 kg. Ideal weight: 73/75.

The estimated calories he intakes before starting the diet: 3800 a day. Calories necessary to keep the excess weight of 90 kg: 3200. Calories necessary to keep the ideal weight of 75 kg: about 2600 (75 kg x 35 = cal. 2600).

Second group - Subject B_1

Woman, height: 1.80 m. Frame: heavy. Weight: 90 kg. Max compatible ideal weight = 75 kg; calories introduced = at least about 3000. Calories necessary to keep the possible ideal weight of 75 kg reached = 2250 (75 kg x 30 cal.) (suggested not more than 1800-2000).

(Diet in common to the 2 subjects B and B_1) - dropping of calories

Weight reached (starting from 90 kg)	Number of kilos lost	Number of treatment days (on average)	Calories of the diet
86	4	20	1600
83	3	10	1200
80	3/2	10	900
77	3/2	10	600
78/77	12/13	50	—-

As an example of a 1600 calorie diet, we have proposed, in the fifth part of this book, the "Health Diet", a hygienic diet preventive of many dismetabolic disease (obesity, gout, hyperuricemia, arteriosclerosis, heart attack, hypercholesterolemia). This diet can be also used as a diet of 2000 and 1600 calories in the stages of subjects B and C. It is also a diet against cancer for its high content in fibers, vitamins and mineral salts.

Rise of calories of subject B – B_1 after the first 50 days of diet Weight reached at the end of 50 days = 78-77 kg

Weight reached (starting again from 78/77)	Number of kilos further lost	Number of permanence days in the different diets	Progressive calories of the diet (going up)
77/76	1	10	from 600 to 900
76/75	1	10	from 900 to 1200
75/74	1-0	10	from 1200 to 1400
73	2/3	30	

The subjects, during the rising of calories in about 4 weeks, not only does not put on weight but on the contrary they lose 2/3 kg more (as normal situation). The dual numbers in this, like in other charts, not only show the variability man/woman, but also the variability of the result inside the same group of people.

I want to make a pause and give in advance, in this part of the book (and not in the F.A.Q.), the answer to a question frequently asked by Italian readers. The seven examples I have chosen among the different ones, to exemplify to the wide public the commonest situations of obesity, does not include purposely the B.M.I, (so-called body mass index). We have also left out the measurement of the wrist, the post scapular skin fold and the distinction between thin and fat mass. The reason is that I consider these aspects too detailed and technical for the wide public[5] who, vice versa, can be bewildered from their principal aims which are to be on a good diet in a good concentration.

Third group - Subject C

Man, height: 1.80 m. Frame: medium. Initial weight: 105 kg. First stage: from 105 to 90 kg. Ideal weight: 75. The estimated calories he intakes before starting the diet: about 4000 - 4500 a day. Calories necessary to keep the excess weight of 105 kg: 3500. Calories necessary to keep the ideal weight:

---

5   Apart from the fact that the knowledge of all these elements does not improve substantially the treatment of obesity beyond a certain limit, do not ever forget that the examples we have outlined refer to hypothetical subjects achieving approximate results. It would be exaggerated then to suppose as to the subjects further data and measurements as if they were in front of us, in person.

about 2500 - 2600 (when he reaches about 75 kg) (suggested not more than 2200 / day).

Between first and second cycle (when his weight is 90) = 2800 /day.

Third group - Subject C₁

Woman, height: 1.80 m. Frame: heavy (or very robust). Weight: about 105 kg. Job: sedentary (or light). The estimated calories she intakes: about 3200-3600. Calories necessary to keep the final ideal weight of 75 kg = about 2250 (after having finished this first cycle and the second one).

(suggested precautionally not more than 1800 - 2000 / day).

First stage: Drop of calories of subjects C-C1 to lose weight from 105 to about 89-90

Weight reached (starting from 105)	Number of kilos lost	Number of treatment days (on average)	Calories of the diet
101	4	20	2000
98	3	10	1600
95	3	10	1200
92	3	10	900
89-90	3-2	10	700
about 89-90	about 16-15	60	-------------

After having finished the first cycle (from 105 to 89-90 kg), a second cycle will be necessary, after a pause of months, to reach the final goal of about 75 kg. It is necessary to start with a diet of at least 2000 calories and finish with that of 700, without following a diet with fewer calories. As to the diets of 1600 and 2000 calories my advice is to use the "Health Diet", described in details in the fifth part.

Michele D'Antoni, MD

First rise of calories of subjects C – C₁ after the first 60 days of diet

Weight reached at the end of 60 days = about 89-90 kg

Weight reached (starting again from 89/90 kg)	Number of kilos lost	Number of permanence days in the different diets	Progressive calories of the diet (going up)
89/90	1-0	7	from 700 to 900
89/90	1-0	7	from 900 to 1200
89/90	1-0	7	from 1200 to 1400
89-90	-	7	from 1600 to 2000
90	0	28	—

The subjects C – C1 during the 4 weeks of rising of calories (especially C1 woman) do not put on weight but do not lose other kilos for the high caloric standard of the diets used during the rise (1200 calories on average), and for the fact to be still very distant from the ideal weight.

The subjects C – C1 have finished their first cycle. After a break of about 3 months, they will start the second cycle (which is identical to that followed by subjects B – B1. The caloric intake in this break will be 2300 calories, subject C1 (woman); 2500-2900 subject C (man).

Second stage: Drop of calories of subjects C-C₁ to lose weight from 90 to about 74

Weight reached (starting again from 90)	Number of kilos lost	Number of treatment days (on average)	Calories of the diet
86	4	20	1600
83	3	10	1200
80	3/2	10	900
77	3/2	10	600
78/77	12/13	50	—

Second rise of subjects C - C₁ after the second stage of the diet
Weight reached at the end of 50 days of the second cycle: 78 - 77

68

Weight reached (starting again from 78/77)	Number of kilos further lost	Number of treatment days	Progressive calories of the diet
77/76	1	10	from 600 to 900
76/75	1	10	from 900 to 1200
75/74	1/0	10	from 1200 to 1600
75/74	2/3	30	------------------

This time the subjects $C - C_1$, in the rising of calories, lose some kilos more and keep the result reached stable. As somebody probably has already noticed the second cycle of the subjects $C - C_1$, coincides exactly with the stages of the two preceding cases B. The subjects C, in fact, are similar to subjects B, but unlike these last ones, are not 15 kg overweight (90 instead of 74-75), but 30 (105 instead of 75). In this case, we are in front of some supposed situations (and real in the same time) which cannot be anymore defined of medium obesity but heavy one. It would be interesting to put forward some other hypothesis. I will be happy and tempted to do, but I do not want to in the interest of the readers. I fear that the excessive exemplifications can at last bewilder them rather than help them having to deal with too many numbers.

In the following pages we will list the menus of 5 main levels *of* calories (1600 - 1400 - 1200 - 900 - 600) which the slimming diets are based on.

As to the diets from 1600 to 2000 calories, it is necessary to follow the "Health Diet" in the two versions: 2000 calories and a little bit reduced, 1600 calories. In relation to the diets of 1400 calories you can elaborate them in a very simple way, by adding, almost daily, to the menu of 1200 calories, 30 gr. of pasta (or rice) in addition to the foreseen 50 gr. (50+30); the same for 50 gr. of bread (30+50) more than the quantity due during the day. For your convenience, some arrows have been inserted in that meals where it is more indicated the addition during the different days of 1200 calories.

For each caloric level, a chart will follow where all the composition of food described in the menu are analyzed in details. We also specify the counting of calories according to sugars, fats or proteins.

From now on, everyone will know not only how many calories a roll contains but also how many grams of the various chemical substances composing it.

For example, the counting of 76 calories introduced with an egg (average weight 50 gr.) is made in the following way:

Proteins: 6.3 gr. multiplied by 4 calories per gram is a total of 25 calories.

Fats: 5.50 gr. multiplied by 9 calories per gram is a total of 50 calories.

Carbohydrates: 0.30 gr. multiplied by 4 calories per gram is a total of 1.2 calories.

Therefore 25+50+1.2 = about 76 calories.

The data related to the ideal weight and height of the seven assumed subjects have been formulated doing a mean of values from different sources and wide personal experience.

The fundamental diets of the Progressive Method

1 OZ = 30 grams
1 Libre = 453 grams

MONDAY

Breakfast
    1 full-fat yogurt (neither low-fat, nor with fruit) 100-120 g
    (or full-fat milk, same quantity)
    1 large and light coffee (as you like also espresso or strong) sweetened
    with 20 g of raw honey
    200 g of fruit as you like (fruit can be eaten for lunch)

Lunch
    Creamed vegetables (asparagus, spinach, and so on) a cup,
    or 200 g boiled carrots, cut into pieces, with lemon
    Oil 10 g (two teaspoons)
    Roast-beef or very lean veal g 100
    2 rusks

Afternoon snack (it can replace dessert for dinner)
    Pineapple or sliced orange 200 g (or other fruit as you like), with some
    natural sugar sprinkled (20 g, two teaspoons), 2 rusks (10 g in total), or
    1 biscuit

Dinner
    Roasted fish 200 g (sword fish) or stewed (sole)
    or oysters (net weight 200 g)
    Oil 10 g
    Boiled string bean 300 g, with lemon, oregano, herbs, parsley
    Bread 60 g
    Ice-cold strawberry-tea, in summer,
    or hot flavored in winter (see page 115)
    Eventually fruit if you did not eat it for breakfast

Logical analysis of Monday's diet

Food and quantity (in gram)	Calories	Proteins (in gram)	Fats (in gram)	Carbohydrates (in gram)	Cholesterol (in mg)
Meat 100 g (roast-beef 100g)	89	20	1	---	68 (x2)
Full-fat yogurt 100-120 g (1 jar)	76	4,2	4,68	4,32	10
Honey 20 g	64	—	—	16	—
Pineapple 200 g	84	1	—	20	—
Fruit 200 g	96	0,6	0,6	22	—
String beans 300 g	56	6,3	0,3	7	—
Bread 60 g/30	160	5,44	0,36	33,6	—
Oil 20 g	180	—	20	—	—
Sole 200 g	172	34	3,4	1,4	114
Sugar 10 g	40	—	—	10	—
Rusks (4) 20 g	76	2,26	0,12	16,5	—
Carrots 200 g	70	1,2	0,54	15,2	—
Total grams (uncooked)		75	31	146	192-260
Total calories of the day /100 730=1400	1163	300 (g 75 x 4 cal)	279 (g 31 x 9 cal)	584 (g 146x4 cal)	
Percentages (optimized)	100%	25.79%	23.98%	50.30%	

Explanation of the charts

I think it right to give straightaway some clarifications to the charts inserted in this chapter and in the next ones. We know that each gram of proteins and sugars develops 4 calories and but each gram of lipids (or fats) develops 9 calories. The total calories, developed in the different food, are obtained therefore by multiplying the number of grams (of each food) by 4

or 9, according to whether we consider proteins (x4), sugars (x4), or fats or lipids (x9). The analytical composition has been calculated doing a mean of values which have been extracted from different sources.
and finally adapted by the author.

Notice: All diets contained in this book have been created exclusively by the Author, and therefore are all original.

Important: the count refers constantly to food weighed always uncooked, and even if precise, you have to consider them in a flexible way, so that you can leave room for minimum changes. If the teaspoon you normally use to measure out honey or sugar, instead of containing exactly 5 g, contains 4.5 or 4, the result is that after 4 times you have eaten 2-4 grams less you will have eaten 8-16 calories less.

Obviously this is not one of the most important factors to pay attention to while following, a slimming treatment.

If you are very gluttonous rand when you open a jar of honey or jam you cannot control yourselves, because instead of eating a few teaspoons you devour half a jar, this is of great importance. The immediate solution in the future is to do without that food and substitute the calories with some other food (for example, more fruit, some more rusks).

The caloric value of all carbohydrates has been rounded off to 4 calories per gram to make the reader get used to the concept that each gram of sugars or carbohydrates develops 4 calories. Actually, just to make an example, the exact calories developed by a gram of sugar are 3.92. However, the exigence to make the reader get used and in some cases remember also the calories of a certain food, has given me the idea to unify the quantities preferably always within the same grams, or multiples: for example, bread always 30+30, fruit 100-200-300, rusks 2-4-6, meat or fish 100-150- 200 gr. and so on.

For this reason, it also necessary, in some cases to round up, while in some other ones, we have left numbers with two decimal figures.

The fruit foreseen refers to that you can find sill year round: apples, pears, pineapples, oranges.

Important: Diabetic subjects, especially if they assume insulin; must consult their personal physician when they go down the 1200 calories level.

However, in summer, it is obvious you can take advantage of fruit in season: cherries, peaches, apricots, unless you do not feel like it. The changes in calories from one kind of fruit to another one are slight, or however not so important to provoke the upsetting of the foreseen total calories of your day.

Remark about the day

Very plain and fresh food, easy to cook. Note in particular the combination of string beans with fish and with the ice-cold tea, which goes along as beverage: it substitutes ice-cold white wine very well.

Very original (since we are speaking about slimming diet) the afternoon snack, very tasty and energetic.

In the successive versions, we propose, day after day, some menus equivalent to the first ones, not only for the quantity of daily calories, but also because proteins, fats and sugars are divided into almost equal percentages.

Of course, we cannot deny that the proposed food are simpler. They do not include, for example, long-drinks and they do not have the fancy that can please us, even if only hinted at.

Creativity has been purposefully reduced to the minimum, in order to avoid transforming these diets into the usual very complicated recipes. Unfortunately, a great part of these publications, which in titles and advertisement promise grandiose novelties to obese people, are reduced at the end to mere cookery. The greatest part of these books could be summed up into two pages (scarcely) which would contain the novelties or the "big secrets" revealed. As to the rest, the pages are a spitted image of the gastronomic encyclopedia, which can be found on the kitchen shelves.

On the contrary, when I read different diet-books from other countries (France, USA, UK, etc.) it seems that the only worry is to make the readers prepare savory dishes, instead of trying to outline a strategy to lose weight with relative caloric levels for the different subjects and a probable result in a given period of time (that is, practically, to fix some slimming schedule, as I have done in this book, let me say for the first time in the world). They concentrate above all on the cooking and ask their readers to dedicate lot of time and attention to the recipe, requiring them to become indirectly skilled cook.

Of course, it is a good feeling to eat savory dishes but it is even better when you can eat a generous meal. Otherwise, if we have to be satisfied with a more modest portion for the time being, this serves as only to open the doors to your ENEMY number one, which is not obesity, but HUNGER!!

It is nonsense saying that you eat little, but "that little I eat is very savory" (and therefore appetizing). This is one of the main traps the person who has to lose weight falls into. It is true obeses are almost always gourmands who love cooking. Just for this reason, it would be better for them to change lifestyle.

I do not want to misuse the famous sentence (also because I disagree) "eating for living and not living for eating" because this could then mean - for example - gulp down into your tummy a certain amount of food and that's it!

As if you took some food and threw it into a bag, without trying to feel that important feelings and emotions the food <u>must transmit</u>.

Changing lifestyle could, on the contrary, mean to get used to eat food which are as savory as simple but above all easy to be found, to be bought, fresh, easy to cook in few minutes, light to digest. They have to leave you enough energy and much free time to dedicate to other activities you like, limiting your time in the kitchen what is strictly necessary, avoiding thus, to make your kitchen a fixed camp.

Think at it: in your house you have the bedroom to sleep; the bathroom to wash yourself; the living room to spend your free time; the kitchen you ought to use only (if you are obese) to cook quickly your food and then to go out, to go to make a walk, by foots or by car or phone to some friends of your either you have family or you are single. American kitchen are very beautiful, but until you will get out from obesity, use them strictly.

Michele D'Antoni, MD

Data in this scheme and the following have been extracted from various sources, and finally, doing a mean of values, adapted by the Author.

DIET of about 1200 cal. (Monday) Main vitamins and mineral salts (in mg.) contained in the diet	Ca	Fe	Na	K	P	Zn	Vit. B1	Vit. A B carotene in µg	Vit. C
Meat gr. 100 (lean)	12	2.3	100	350	200	---	0.07	---	---
Yogurt 120 gr.	180	---	70	200	120	---	---	245	---
French beans gr. 300	120	2.9	6	840	48	---	0.21	750	48
Carrots gr. 200	88	1.4	100	480	80	0.8	0.08	14000	8
Rusks gr. 20	10	0.6	---	---	110	---	0.4	---	---
Bread gr. 60	38	0.4	450	100	80	0.5	0.2	---	---
Sole gr. 200 (preferably oysters)	280	12	980	520	540	12/50	---	---	---
Pineapple gr. 200	24	0.4	---	500	20	0.4	0.16	120	34
Fruit gr. 200 (orange)	50	0.4	0.6	400	44	0.4	0.04	852	100
Total values of Monday	802	20.4	1700	3390	1236	13/40	1.22	15967	190
Total values of daily requirement	600/800	10/18	2200	3100	1000	7/10	0.8/1	4200	60

N.B. Values are expressed in milligrams, except Vit. A in µg (micrograms)
Values of vitamin A are expressed in carotene-B.

Factor of conversion: 1 µg of R:E (retinol equivalent) = 6 µg of B-carotene.

76

Alternative version of Monday

Meals and foods proposed	Calories	Cholesterol
Breakfast Coffee Skimmed milk g. 150 Sugar g 10 Total calories 1 empty croissant	-- 54 0 94	3
Lunch Mozzarella cheese gr. 60 Boiled vegetables as you like g 300- Spinach Sliced tomato g 200 Bread g 60 Oil to season g 10 Pear g. 200 Total calories	152 60 40 160 60 85 547	57
Dinner Stewed dried beans (cooked with small onions and tomato) g 100 Parmesan g 10 Azure fish g 100-120 cooked as you like Bread g 30 Apple g 100 Total calories	264 37 135 80 45 561	9,5 85,5
Total calories (+ croissant) = 1400	**1202**	**155 mg.**

TUESDAY

Breakfast
    Skimmed milk 200 g sweetened with 20 g of raw honey
    1 coffee
    Fruit 100 g as you like
    2 rusks with 20 g jam

Lunch
    2 boiled artichokes (200 g totally) or boiled string bean 300 gr., with lemon, oregano, herbs, parsley.
    Oil 5 g
    Cooked ham g 50
    Bread g 30
    Fruit g 200 (bananas g 100)

Afternoon snack
    1 apple of 100 g cooked in the oven, or a glass of cocktail rosé (see recipe on page 122)

Dinner
    50 g tagliatelle, spaghetti with peeled tomatoes
    before serving add a teaspoon of oil, one of grated cheese and a pinch of salt.
    Roasted veal (very lean) g 150
    100 g carrots finely grated
    Orange g 200 (or pineapple, same quantity) cut into slices around the meat, as
    a garnish

If you do not want to eat pasta, you can use rice or lentils in the same quantity. You can replace raw honey with the normal one or a couple of sachets of sweetener. The two artichokes can be substituted with 300 g of string beans frozen too, or with asparagus, same quantity.

If you do not eat the afternoon snack, the ingredients of the cocktail rosé can be used in a different way: the orange (g 100) which contains for our convenience also half lemon, can be drunk any time during the day or be added to that of the evening; carrots (g 100) can be vice versa eaten for lunch, together with artichokes and ham.

Logical analysis of Tuesday's diet

Food and quantity (in gram)	Calories	Proteins (in gram)	Fats (in gram)	Carbohydrates (in gram)	Cholesterol (in mg)
Cooked ham g 50	206	10,75	18,15	—	32
Skimmed milk g 200	72	7,2	0,1	10,6	4
2 rusks	38	—	—	—	---
Honey g 20	64	—	—	16	—
Jam g 20	38	—	—	13	—
Orange g. 300	138	4	0,6	29	—
Fruit (tot.) g 300	128	0,9	1,1	28,5	—
50 g di tagliatelle	190	5	0,42	40	—
Carrots g 100	35	1,15	—	7,8	—
Bread g. 30/ Bread g. 60	80	2,7	0,18	16,8	—
Oil g 10	90	—	10	—	—
Veal g 150	134	31	1,1	—	100
Artichokes g. 200	45	5,4	0,4	5	---
Total grams (uncooked)		68	32.05	174	136
Total calories of the day Bread gr. 60 = 1400	1256	272 (g 68x4 cal)	288 (g 32 x 9 cal)	696 (g 174x4 cal)	
Percentages (optimized)	100%	21.6%	23%	55.3%	

Remark about the day

This is a classical example of a balanced slimming diet: total daily calories = 1256; percentages of optimal sugars and proteins (55% and 22%). The breakfast is fresh, energetic and nourishing (200 calories). Classical dinner. Original lunch with artichokes which make the ham lighter.

This diet has been proposed because the food is simple, ready to cook. This is very suitable for a day like Tuesday which is full of engagement

Data in this scheme and the following have been extracted from various sources, and finally, doing a mean of values, adapted by the Author.

DIET of about 1200 cal. (Tuesday) Main vitamins and mineral salts (in mg.) contained in the diet	Ca	Fe	Na	K	P	Zn	Vit. B1	Vit. A B carotene in µg	Vit. C
Cooked ham gr. 50	5	2.0	1000	150	80	1.8	0.30	Tr	Tr
Skimmed milk gr. 200	240	0.06	100	270	180	0.5	0.08	Tr	Tr
Oranges gr. 300	150	0.6	6	675	24	0.3	0.09	1300	150
Fruit (tot) gr. 200	60	1.4	12	260	170	---	0.06	Tr	Tr
Banana g. 100	7	0.8	1	350	28	0.2	0.06	270	7
Tagliatelle g.50	8	1	13	140	120	1.3	0.10	0	0
Carrots g. 100	45	0.6	50	240	40	0.4	0.08	6.800	4
Bread g. 30 (like rolls)	18	0.3	220	50	40	0.25	0.1	---	---
Veal (lean meat) g. 150	18	2.8	150	520	300	1.4	0.2	---	---
Artichokes gr. 200 (net)	180	2	260	720	138	1.4	0.9	216	24
Total values of Tuesday	720	1820	1820	3375	1120	7.5	1.9	8586	185
Total values of daily requirement	600/800	2200	2200	3100	1000	7/10	0.8/1	4200	60

N.B. Values are expressed in milligrams, except Vit. A in µg (micrograms)

Values of vitamin A are expressed in carotene-B.

Factor of conversion: 1 µg of R:E (retinol equivalent) = 6 µg of B-carotene.

Alternative version of Tuesday

Meals and foods proposed	Calories	Cholesterol
Breakfast Skimmed milk g. 300 Tea (or coffee) + 2 rusks Sugar g 10 + jam g 10 Total calories	36 38 80 154	2
Lunch Lean fish (sole) g. 200 Lettuce or raw tomatoes g 200 Oil to season g 10 Bread-sticks g 20 (or bread g. 30) Pear g. 100 Total calories	168 40 90 80 85 463	114
Dinner g 50 tagliatelle, spaghetti with peeled tomato Grilled beef not very lean g 100 (lipids 15%) Boiled vegetables (zucchini, carrots, spinach, onions) g. 200 Bread g 30/30 Apple or orange according to the season g 200 Total calories	190 210 50 80 80-90 610	68
Total calories (+ 30 + 50)=1400	**1227**	**186 ma.**

N. B. To bring all diets from 1200 to 1400 calories, it is necessary to add the quantities with the (+) sign to the food already listed, ex. Tuesday (alternative version):

Calories foreseen = 1227 cal. (about)

In addition + 30 g bread = 75 cal.

In addition + 30 g rice + or spaghetti or beans = 108 cal.

= 1410 cal. (about)

WEDNESDAY

Breakfast
>   1 glass of American-style-shake (see recipe on page 122)
>   or g 200 skimmed milk
>   1 coffee
>   1 biscuit g 10
>   Raw honey g 20 (or sugar or jam same quantity)

Lunch
>   1 hard-boiled egg (or soft-boiled)
>   boiled spinach with lemon g 300
>   Oil g 5
>   Bread g 30
>   Flavored tea, hot

Afternoon snack
>   A glass of cold milk g 200

Dinner
>   Stewed beef g 100 (not very fat)
>   Boiled lentils g 50 or dried beans g 60 or the same amount of calories of frozen beans with tomato, onion, garlic, and so on
>   Aromatic herbs
>   Oil g 5
>   Bread g 30
>   Fruit g 200 as you like (or 1 glass of apple juice flavored with cinnamon)

Logical analysis of Wednesday's diet

Food and quantity (in gram)	Calories	Proteins (in gram)	Fats (in gram)	Carbohydrates (in gram)	Cholesterol (in mg)
Skimmed milk g. 200	85	0,6	0,8	19	—
Apples g. 200	96	0,6	0,6	22	—
American-style-shake or 1	82	1.2	0.5	18.2	—
glass of cold milk	64	—	—	16	—
Honey g 20	39	0,65	0,8	7,3	—
1 biscuit g 10	76	6,3	5,6	0,1	210
1 egg g 50	95	10,2	2,1	8,9	—
Spinach g 300	160	5,4	0,36	33,6	—
Bread g 60/40	159	12,5	1,25	24,5	—
Lentils g 50/30	19	1	—	3,75	—
Peeled tomato g 100	13	0,5	—	2,75	—
Onion g 50	90	—	10	—	—
Raw oil g 10 (+10)	170	20	10	——————	68
Beef (not very fat) g 100					
Total grams		58.95	32	156	278
Total calories of the day /40/30=1400	1148	236 (g 59 x 4 cal)	288 (g 32 x 9 cal)	624 (g 156x4 cal)	
Percentages (optimized)	100%	20.55%	15.08%	54.35%	

Remark about the day

Food to be eaten in your home both for the frugality (the egg and the spinach), and for the way to cook them. It is pretty sure you cannot find anywhere the stewed beef and the lentils cooked with little salt, healthy onions and peeled tomato without oil (only 5 g). Not to mention the tasty flavored apple juice. Nobody in the world, or almost, knows about it.

Data in this scheme and the following have been extracted from various sources, and finally, doing a mean of values, adapted by the Author.

DIET of about 1200 cal. (Wednesday) Main vitamins and mineral salts (in mg.) contained in the diet	Ca	Fe	Na	K	P	Zn	Vit. B1	Vit. A B carotene in µg	Vit. C
Fruit gr. 400 (tot) (apples, pears)	160	2.4	24	520	340	4.8	0.8	---	---
Grapefruit (orange) gr. 200	100	0.4	4	250	16	0.2	0.06	850	100
1 egg (gr. 50 on average)	24	1.2	70	70	105	0.7	0.6	660	0
Spinachs gr. 300	230	8.7	300	1500	186	1.2	1.6	8.700	162
Bread gr. 60	36	0.4	466	100	66	0.5	0.02	0	0
Lentils gr. 50	80	6	50	368	170	1.6	0.1	60	3
Peeled tomatoes gr. 100 (ripe)	8	0.3	8	200	20	---	0.03	2600	25
Small onions gr. 50	25	0.4	6	115	24	---	0.05	Tr	3
Half lean meat gr. 100	10	2.1	100	350	180	1.3	0.1	---	---
Total values of Wednesday	60	22	1030	3473	1002	11.6	2.7	12870	283
Total values of daily requirement	600/800	10/18	2200	3100	1000	7/10	0.8/1	4200	60

N.B. Values are expressed in milligrams, except Vit. A in µg (micrograms)

Values of vitamin A are expressed in carotene-B.

Factor of conversion: 1 µg of R:E (retinol equivalent) = 6 µg of B-carotene.

Alternative version of Wednesday

Meals and foods proposed	Calories	Cholesterol
Breakfast Orange juice or skimmed milk g 250 2 rusks 1 coffee Jam g 10 Sugar g 10 Total calories	90 38 38 40 206	
Lunch Mozzarella cheese g. 100 Tomato g 200 Oil g 10 Bread g. 30 / 50 Fruit g. 100 Total calories	250 40 90 80 45-50 505	95
Dinner Pasta (spaghetti) g 50 / 30 Peeled tomato g 100 Chicken breast g 100 (or turkey) Bread sticks g 20 (or bread g 30) Fruit (apples, pears g 100) Total calories	190 20 90 80 45-50 (on average) 429	67
Total daily calories (+ 30 + 50)=1400	**1139**	**162 mg.**

THURSDAY

Breakfast
> Skimmed milk g 200
> 1 coffee
> Raw honey g 15
> 1 fruit g 100 (orange) at about 11 a.m.
> 1 small fruit fancy cake 20 - 30 g as you like

Lunch
> Smashed potatoes g 200 (or potatoes with butter, same quantity;
> to prepare them, use 10 g butter and 10 g parmesan)
> Sword fish with orange 100 g (or grilled veal, same quantity)
> Grapefruit cocktail (see recipe on page 122)
> 1 glass (total g 200), or 1 fruit as you like g 200

Afternoon snack
> Fruit g 200 (we recommend 1 pear cut into pieces g 150, strawberries or
> raspberries g 50, g 5 honey or sugar, lemon)

Dinner
> Cow mozzarella cheese g 100
> Sliced tomatoes g 300 with oregano, lemon
> Bread 30 g
> Fruit g 100 (banana)

N. B. If you want to, you can change lunch with dinner, (as usual, if it is easier for you to prepare for dinner the food proposed for the lunch, and vice versa).

Logical analysis of Thursday's diet

Food and quantity (in gram)	Calories	Proteins (in gram)	Fats (in gram)	Carbohydrates (in gram)	Cholesterol (in mg)
Milk, g. 200	72	7	0.1	10.6	—
Honey g 20 (eventually with sugar included)	64	—	—	16	—
1 small fruit fancy cake/1	80	2	0.45	18	—
Fruit g 300	128	0.9	1.2	28.5	—
Fruit g 300 (orange) (or grapefruit cocktail)	137	4	0.6	29	´
Potatoes g 200	164	4	—	36	--
Butter g 10	72	—	8	—	29
Parmesan g 10	37	3.5	2.5	0.3	10
Grilled sword fish g 100	137	19	5	4	70
Cow mozzarella cheese g 100	246	20	16		100
Tomato g 300	57	3	—	11.25	—
Bread g 30/50	80	2.7	0.18	16.8	68
Total grams		66	34	176	209
Total calories of the day /80/50=1400	**1274**	**264** (g 66 x 4 cal)	**306** (g 34 x 9 cal)	**704** (g 176x4 cal)	
Percentages (optimized)	**100%**	**20.75%**	**24%**	**55.25%**	

Remark about the day

Some more society remarks start peeping out, especially more frequently until Sunday. Breakfasts are always remarkable, nourishing and energetic. The afternoon snack is delicious, by now you are already spoiled! Try to imagine your friends' faces when you tell them your breakfast and afternoon snack include honey and sugar! Just think about what they would do to include them in their daily menu! But they cannot, obviously, because your afternoon snack contains only 150 calories, after all. On the contrary, they are part of the large group who cannot swallow anything without oil and salt. Therefore, if they to eat three teaspoons more, they have to give up the afternoon snack

Data in this scheme and the following have been extracted from various sources, and finally, doing a mean of values, adapted by the Author.

DIET of about 1200 cal. (Thursday) Main vitamins and mineral salts (in mg.) contained in the diet	Ca	Fe	Na	K	P	Zn	Vit. B1	Vit. A B carotene in µg	Vit. C
Milk gr. 200	240	0.03	100	270	180	0.5	---	---	---
Fruit gr. 300 (raspberries, strawberries, pears)	90	2.1	18	530	500	---	0.08	100	75
Potatoes gr. 200	20	6	4	1070	54	---	0.4	---	---
Sword-fish (or azure fish) gr. 200	70	0.8	110	430	280	0.4	0.2	---	---
Parmesan gr. 10	130	0.07	51	10	24	0.2	0.06	17	---
Banana gr. 100	7	0.8	1	350	28	0.2	0.06	270	7
Fruits gr. 200 (orange or grapefruit for the cocktail)	50	0.2	20	400	48	0.1	0.03	426	50
Mozzarella cheese gr. 100	480	0.3	137	37	200	4.7	0.07	1200	---
Tomatoes (ripe) gr. 300	18	0.2	4	200	35	0.2	0.04	5000	3
Bread gr. 30	18	0.2	233	50	33	0.25	0.01	---	---
Carrots gr. 80		0.2	4	200	35	0.2	0.04	5000	3
Total values of Thursday	1152	11.4	688	4277	1552	7	1	9413	213
Total values of daily requirement	600/800	10/18	2200	3100	1000	7/10	0.8/1	4200	60

N.B. Values are expressed in milligrams, except Vit. A in µg (micrograms)

Values of vitamin A are expressed in carotene-B.

Factor of conversion: 1 µg of R:E (retinol equivalent) = 6 µg of B-carotene.

Alternative version of Thursday

Meals and foods proposed	Calories	Cholesterol
Breakfast Coffee 2 rusks Skimmed milk g 200 (or 1 full-fat yogurt 120 g) Butter g 10 Sugar g 10 Total calories	— 38 73 70 40 221	 4 25
Lunch Cooked ham g 50 Boiled broccoli g 200 Lemon juice as you like Bread g. 60 Fresh pineapple g. 200 or fruit in season Total calories	 206 40 --- 160 106 (on average) 512	 32
Dinner Boiled lentils/beans g 50 / 30 Oil about 5 g Roasted chicken breast g 150 (or turkey) Lemon as you like Lettuce g 50 1 pear g 200 Bread 30/50 Total calories	 182 45 150 -- 10 85 80 550	 67
Total daily calories (+ 90 + 50)=1400	**1285**	**128 mg.**

FRIDAY

Breakfast[1]
>1 yogurt g 100 (we recommend to eat the full-fat
>one, as the low-fat or with fruit do not contain many active principles)
>or fruit fancy cake g 20-30
>1 coffee sweetened with 20 g of raw honey
>1 fruit 100 g (persimmons)

Lunch
>Boiled fish g 200 (small cuttlefish, shrimps)
>Or same quantity, roasted squid, or oysters
>2 potato milk croquettes (or potato g 200 with butter)
>Fruit g 100 (grapes)

Dinner
>Grilled minced meat[2], g 150 (two meatballs)
>Tomato g 300 (or lettuce)
>Lemon juice
>Bread 30 g
>Fruit g 100 (peaches)

---

1 Yogurt can be replaced with 100 g milk (full-fat, too). If you do not eat the fruit (g 100) and the honey (g 20), you can have a small fruit fancy cake 20-30 g. Please, pay attention: you can have only one! If you think, you cannot manage to be satisfied with a single one, in this case forget them...and do not let them come into your house. Nobody thinks we have to act the heroes! The same is for the jar of honey: if you think it can change into an irresistible temptation, just use plain sugar.

2 As minced meat use only lean veal of first quality. Mix only some tablespoons of milk, egg and the parmesan foreseen (g 20). For the croquettes at lunch use some milk and 10 g butter.

Logical analysis of Friday's diet

Food and quantity (in gram)	Calories	Proteins (in gram)	Fats (in gram)	Carbohydrates (in gram)	Cholesterol (in mg)
Fruit g 300	128	0.9	1.2	28,5	—
Parmesan g 20	74	7	4.9	0,6	20
Tomato g 300	63	3	0.65	11,25	—
Bread g 30/50	80	2.7	0.18	16,8	—
Meat g 150	135	30.8	1.3	—	100
Butter g 10	74	—	8.2	—	25
Full-fat yogurt g 120 (+1 in the afternoon)	76	4.1	4.68	4,32	10
Honey g 20	64	-	—	16	
Potatoes g 200	162	4	0.3	36	
Sole g 200	166	33.7	2.8	1,5	114
Milk g 100	36	3.5	0.2	5	10
1 egg	76	6.3	5.6	0,1	
Total grams		**96**	**30**	**120**	**179**
Total calories of the day /80/50=1400	**1134**	**384** (g 96 x 4 cal)	**270** (g 30 x 9 cal)	**480** (g 120x4 cal)	
Percentages (optimized)	**100%**	**33.86%**	**23.80%**	**42.32%**	

Remark about the day

We start with some menus which can be easily ordered also in a restaurant, if you are out for your meals. The fish with croquettes is very typical and can be substituted with plain steamed potatoes.

Very easy also the cooking of the grilled minced beef.

If you eat out, ask to use little flour for the preparation of meat and croquettes. For both menus we have used not more than one egg.

Data in this scheme and the following have been extracted from various sources, and finally, doing a mean of values, adapted by the Author.

DIET of about 1200 cal. (Friday) Main vitamins and mineral salts (in mg.) contained in the diet	Ca	Fe	Na	K	P	Zn	Vit. B1	Vit. A B carotene in µg	Vit. C
Fruit gr. 100 (bananas)	7	0.8	1	350	28	0.2	0.06	270	17
(grapes)	27	0.4	2	285	4	0.1	0.1	23	4
(persimmons)	8	0.3	25	87	16	0.1	0.02	1422	23
Parmesan gr. 20	268	0.7	87	20	180	0.1	Tr.	19	---
Tomatoes (preferably lettuce) gr. 300	150	2.4	150	730	99	0.6	0.05	1574	18
Bread gr. 30	18	0.3	220	50	40	0.25	0.1	---	---
Meat (lean) g. 150	20	2	150	520	300	---	1.2	---	---
Butter gr. 10	20	0.8	20	26	20	0.1	0.1	60	2
Full-fat yogurt (120 gr.)	170	0.1	60	200	120	0.01	0.06	280	1
Potatoes gr. 200	10	1.2	14	1040	108	0.6	0.2	88	30
Fish gr. 200 (oysters)	280	12	980	520	540	12-50	---	450	---
Skimmed milk gr. 100	120	0.3	50	270	180	0.5	0.08	Tr.	Tr.
Total values of Friday	1082	21	1757	4098	1635	14-52	1.9	4190	95
Total values of daily requirement	600/800	10/18	2200	3100	1000	7/10	0.8/1	4200	60

N.B. Values are expressed in milligrams, except Vit. A in µg (micrograms)

Values of vitamin A are expressed in carotene-B.

Factor of conversion: 1 µg of R:E (retinol equivalent) = 6 µg of B-carotene.

Alternative version of Friday

Meals and foods proposed	Calories	Cholesterol
Breakfast		
Full-fat yogurt g 120 (or skimmed milk g 200)	72	10
2 rusks	38	
Jam g 10	40	
1 coffee with sweetener (saccharine)	-	
Total calories	150	
Lunch		
Azure fish g 100 - 120 cooked as you like	140	100
Boiled potatoes g 300 (seasoned with lemon)	240	
Bread g 30 / 50	80	
Fruit in season (orange)	50	
Total calories	430	
Dinner		
Tagliatelle or rice g 50 /30	194	
Peeled tomato g 100	20	
Boiled vegetables (spinach) g 300	60	
1 hard-boiled egg	152	210
Bread sticks g 20 (or bread g 30 / 50)	80	
Oil 2 teaspoons	90	
Lemon as you like	--	
Total calories	596	
Total daily calories (+ 50 + 50 + 30=1400)	**1176**	**320 mg.**

SATURDAY

Breakfast
 Strawberry milk shake (see recipe on page 122) or skimmed milk g 200
 Apple g 100
 Raw honey g 20
 1 coffee

Lunch
 Fried newborn fish balls (sardines) g 150, or two frozen fish sticks fried
 Spinach with lemon or raw g 200
 2 rusks 10 g
 Fruit 100 g as you like (grapes)

Dinner
 Dried beans (stewed with small onions and tomato) g 100
 (pr spaghetti g 70 with tomato (g 100)
 1 teaspoon of grated cheese (g 10)
 Roasted chicken breast g 100 (or turkey)
 2 leaves of green salad
 Fruit g 100 (persimmons)
 2 rusks g 10

Logical analysis of Saturday's diet

Food and quantity (in gram)	Calories	Proteins (in gram)	Fats (in gram)	Carbohydrates (in gram)	Cholesterol (in mg)
Milk g 200	72	7.2	0.1	10.6	4
Honey g 20 / 1 croissant	64	—	—	16	—
Fruit g 300	128	0.9	1.2	28.5	—
Fish g 150	157	9.8	12.7	0.8	85 .
Peeled tomato g 100	18	1	—	3.5	—
Butter g 10	75	—	8.3	—	25
Flour g 20	67	2.38	0.33	13.68	—
Fennel g 200	18	2.4	—	2	—
Parmesan g 10	37	3.5	2.5	0.3	10
4 rusks / 4	76	2.26	0.27	16.6	—
Spaghetti (beans) g 70	264	7	0.5	55	—
Chicken breast g 100 (turkey)	97	22.2	0.9	—	67
Total grams		**56.54**	**26.72**	**152.28**	**191**
Total calories of the day **1 croissant /4 fette=1400**	1073,16	226.16 (g 56.54 x 4 cal)	238 (g 26.52 x 9 cal)	609 (g 152.28x4 cal)	
Percentages (optimized)	100%	21%	22.18%	56.75%	

Remark about the day

This day is composed of food which can be easily found in restaurants.

When the dessert is served, we advise you, if you are with other people, to leave the table and phone to your best friend. There is no point in "taking only a bite of it". You will suffer without any reason, by seeing the other who stuff themselves, inducing you to d into temptation, because of their nightmare: you can resist and they cannot.

In addition, that "little bit" you desperately try to make it last, will ruin all the calculations of calories which we have tried hard to do exactly on these charts.

Data in this scheme and the following have been extracted from various sources, and finally, doing a mean of values, adapted by the Author.

DIET of about 1200 cal. (Saturday) Main vitamins and mineral salts (in mg.) contained in the diet	Ca	Fe	Na	K	P	Zn	Vit. B1	Vit. A B carotene in µg	Vit. C
Milk gr. 200 + 200	80	4.0	200	540	360	1	0.12	Tr.	Tr.
Fruit gr. 100 (persimmons)	8	0.3	25	87	16	0.1	0.1	1422	23
gr. 150 (grapes)	27	0.4	2	427	4	0.1	0.1	23	6
gr. 100 (bananas)	7.0	0.8	1	350	28	0.2	0.6.	270	17
Fish gr. 150 (sole)	18	0.16	178	445	300	0.3	0.1	Tr.	0
Peeled tomatoes gr. 100	9	0.2	9	230	24	0.1	Tr.	2400	18
Butter gr. 10	2.5	---	0.7	0.10	0.16	Tr.	---	558	0
Fennel gr. 200 (zucchinis)	90	0.8	8	400	78	2.87	0.04	4	24
Parmesan gr. 10	116	0.07	60	100	67	---	0.03	223	0
4 rusks	20	07	---	---	---	---	---	0	0
Pasta (spaghetti) gr. 70	12	1	20	200	120	1.3	0.3	0	0
Chicken breast gr. 100	10	---	67	325	214	0.7	0.08	0	0.
Total values of Saturday	800	8.43	570	3012	1211	6.57	1.43	4900	89
Total values of daily requirement	600/800	10/18	2200	3100	1000	7/10	0.8/1	4200	60

N.B. Values are expressed in milligrams, except Vit. A in µg (micrograms)

Values of vitamin A are expressed in carotene-B.

Factor of conversion: 1 µg of R:E (retinol equivalent) = 6 µg of B-carotene.

Alternative version of Saturday

Meals and foods proposed	Calories	Cholesterol
Breakfast		
1 coffee	0	
Orange or grapefruit juice g 200	90	
2 rusks	38	
lam g.20/20	60	
Total calories	188	
Lunch		
Vegetable purée g 200	40	90
Stracchino cheese g 100 (or fontina g 70)	250	
Bread g. 30/50	80	
1 apple g 200 (banana g 100)	90	
Total calories	460	114
Dinner		
Azure fish g 100/120 cooked as you like	160	25
Spinach g 300	60	
Butter g 10	74	
Bread sticks g 20 (or bread g 30)	80	
Fresh pineapple or fruit in season g 200	90/100 (on average)	
Total calories	464	
Total daily calories (+20+10+60=1400)	**1112**	**229 mg.**

SUNDAY

Breakfast
>1 large and light coffee sweetened with 10 g of raw honey
>skimmed milk 200 g and coffee

Lunch
>Two toasted sandwiches with ricotta cheese and spinach[3]
>Parma ham g 50
>Cantaloupe melon g 300
>American-style shake (see recipe on page 122) 1 glass,
>or 1 fruit juice as you like

Dinner
>Lean veal g 200
>Boiled asparagus or broccoli g 200
>2 rusks
>Orange g 100
>Flavoured or mint tea.

---

3   You can prepare the sandwiches with 100 g ricotta cheese and 50 g of boiled spinach. Add
     a teaspoon of butter. Fill in the sandwiches with this cream and toast them in the toaster
     or in the oven until golden.
     Alternately, you can have also two toasted sandwiches with 100 g mozzarella cheese (or
     50 g slice of processes cheese) and 50 g tomato.

Logical analysis of Sunday's diet

Food and quantity (in gram)	Calories	Proteins (in gram)	Fats (in gram)	Carbohydrates (in gram)	Cholesterol (in mg)
4 slices of tin loaf g 70	180	2.4	1.5	39.2	
Ricotta cheese g 100	184	4.8	16.14	4.9	32
Spinach g 50	15	1.7	0.21	1.5	—
Parma ham g. 50	179	11.1	15	—	45
Cantaloupe melon g 300	65	1	0.6	13.7	—
Lean veal or beef loin g 200	180	40	2	0.82	145
Orange + lemon for dinner and American-style shake g 300	134	3	0.6	29	—
Skimmed milk g 200	85	0.6	0.6	19	—
Asparagus g 200	58	7	0.4	6.6	—
2 rusks /2	40	1.13	0.3	8.4	----
Total grams		**72.73**	**37.35**	**123.12**	**222**
Total calories of the day 2/200=1400	**1119.55**	**290.92** (g 72.73 x 4 cal)	**336.15** (g 37.35 x 9 cal)	**492.48** (g 123.12x4 cal)	
Percentages (optimized)	**100%**	**26%**	**30%**	**42.32%**	

Remark about the day

We have thought it more advisable to have toasted sandwiches for lunch, because this kind of food cheers up and you can also invite friends. By the way, remember to prepare more than two each, because among your friends, it is pretty sure they will eat more than the recommended quantity. Unless you will have to eat yourself those which are left!

Data in this scheme and the following have been extracted from various sources, and finally, doing a mean of values, adapted by the Author.

DIET of about 1200 cal. (Sunday) Main vitamins and mineral salts (in mg.) contained in the diet	Ca	Fe	Na	K	P	Zn	Vit. B1	Vit. A B carotene in µg	Vit. C
Skimmed milk gr. 200	240	0.06	100	270	180	0.5	0.08	Tr.	Tr.
Fresh tuna (Sword-fish)	76	2.6	84	---	528	1	0.32	2.700	Tr.
Potatoes gr. 200	10	1.2	14	1040	108	0.6	0.2	38	30
Bread gr. 60	36	0.3	440	100	80	0.5	0.2.	---	---
Orange gr. 200	100	0.4	6	400	44	0.4	0.04	852	100
Mozzarella cheese (cow) gr. 70	403	0.2	100	28	150	4	0.05	720	---
Zucchinis gr. 300	63	1.5	1	630	195	0.6	1.2	1110	33
Bread gr. 30	18	0.15	220	50	40	0.25	0.1	---	---
Fruit gr. 200 (apricots)	48	1	Tr.	640	32	0.2	0.06	4.320	26
Total values of Sunday	994	7.41	967	3158	1355	8.05	2.25	9700	192
Total values of daily requirement	600/800	10/18	2200	3100	1000	7/10	0.8/1	4200	60

N.B. Values are expressed in milligrams, except Vit. A in µg (micrograms)

Values of vitamin A are expressed in carotene-B.

Factor of conversion: 1 µg of R:E (retinol equivalent) = 6 µg of B-carotene.

Alternative version of Sunday

Meals and foods proposed	Calories	Cholesterol
Breakfast		
Large light coffee or tea	72	4
Skimmed milk g. 200	40	
Sugar g.10	80	
1 fruit fancy cake (+1)		
Total calories	192	
Lunch		
Grilled sword fish (or dentex or tuna) g 200	260	140
Boiled or steamed potatoes g 200	164	
Oil g 10	90	
Lemon as you like	--	
Bread sticks g 20 (or bread g 30)	80	
Orange g 200	90	
Total calories	684	
Dinner		
Cow mozzarella cheese g 70 - tomato	166	66
Boiled zucchini g 300	60	
Lemon as you like	--	
Bread g 30/50	80	
1 apple g 200	90	
Total calories	396	
Total daily calories (+50 + 1 cake=1400)	**1272**	**210 mg.**

The diets with a more specific caloric level (900-800 kilo-calories)

900 daily calories

This diet is fundamental for the Progressive Method. It represents, in fact, a passage of great importance, which you reach after different days of richer diets.

We could define it:

- *Normocarbohydratic* because carbohydrates, even if reduced in grams, are still contained in the ideal percentage (about 50%). I have decided to keep them constantly, not taking into consideration the opinions of those who think it is better to abolish them if you want to lose weight. We are speaking of top-class sugars, that is those recommended by the Senate of USA like raw honey, wholemeal bread, fruit, milk, vegetables, pulses, starches;

- *hyperproteic* in a relative and wide sense because proteins are as many (68 grams) as those which an adult weighing 70 kg who does not follow any diet should intake. They make the percentage raise from 12 to 30%, in respect to the global diet;

- *hypolipidic,* that is with a low content in fats. They should be, for an adult of about 70 kg, 70 g a day, and on the contrary they are 22 g all together. In percentage, however, they are the optimal quantity (21%). In order not to confuse you, it will be better if you had a look to the foreword where I speak about the optimal proportions of a normal diet;

- *hypocaloric* since the total calories are inferior to the normal ones.

Menu of the 900 calorie diet

Breakfast

> Orange or grapefruit juice g 200
> 1 full-fat yogurt (neither low-fat, nor with fruit) g 100 or semi-skimmed milk g 200
> Wholemeal bread g 50
> Jam g 10
> 1 coffee sweetened with 10 g of raw honey

Lunch

Lean veal g 150, or grilled lean fish g 150

Vegetables g 200-300 (if boiled choose among eggplants, broccoli; if raw, choose among carrots, tomatoes, lettuce seasoned with little oil, oregano. and lemon as you like, just a pinch of salt)

2 rusks g 10

1 coffee (preferably decaffeinated) sweetened with a teaspoon of raw honey

Dinner

Vegetables (lettuce, zucchini, spinach) cooked or soup as you like, or consommé g 300-400;

low-fat cheese (fontina, Bel Paese) g 50

or very lean meat or fish 130-140 g

or mozzarella cheese g 30 and 1 hard or soft boiled egg

with oregano and lemon (only 1 day out of 4);

2 rusks g 10;

Fresh fruit g 100 (or stewed string beans g 200-300)

If you do not eat up the nourishing breakfast in the morning, you can leave something for the afternoon snack, eventually along with a cup of tea or coffee which, as we already know, do not contain calories and therefore do not change the calorie counting. If you do not want to have breakfast at all, we have left 1/3 of calories (330) which we can use in different ways. You can find different alternative versions in the following pages.

Logical analysis of the chemical composition of the 900 calorie diet

Food and quantity (in gram)	Calories	Proteins (in gram)	Carbohydrates (in gram)	Fats (in gram)	Cholesterol (in mg)
Citrus fruit juice g 200	91	3.4	19.3	—	
Full-fat Yogurt g 120	76	4.8	4.32	4.48	10
Wholemeal bread g 50	118	3.8	24.2	0.68	
Jam g 10	28	—	7		
Honey g15	48	—	12		
Meat or fish g 150	135	31	—	1.2	100
Fruit g.100/String beans g 300	48/60	0.3	11	0.3	
Rusks g 20	76	2.1	16.6	0.12	
[Meat or fish g 150] Mozzarella cheese g 70	172	[30]* 13.35	0.4	13	66.5
Eggplants g 100	16	1	2.6	0.2	
Zucchini g 200	22	2.6	2.6	0.2	
Lettuce g 100	20	1.8	2.2	0.4	
Spinach g 100	31	3.4	2.8	0.7	
Carrots g 50	19	0.57	3.8	0.15	
Total grams		68 [85]*	108.82	21.43	176.5
Daily total calories	900	272.48 (g 68.12x4 cal)	435.28 (g 108x4 cal)	192.87 (g 21.43x9 cal)	
Percentages (optimized)	100%	30.27%	48.33%	21.43%	

Remark about the diet

A very rich breakfast, equivalent to about 1/3 of the total calories. You will be not very hungry and tired at lunchtime. Very light lunch and however nourishing.

Dinner is also well balanced and follows the same principles. Ideal for an early morning. You will sleep well and when you get up in the morning, you will find a nourishing breakfast waiting for you. If vice versa you have lost this habit, or you never had it, you can leave the food for the afternoon snack, or, in case you do not have it, a fair dish of starchy food, which will normalize one of the two meals.

Data in this scheme and the following have been extracted from various sources, and finally, doing a mean of values, adapted by the Author.

900 calorie diet	K	P	Ca	Vit. A	Vit C	Fe	Na	Zn	Vit. B1
Oranges gr. 200	400	44	100	426	50	0.2	2	0.1	0.03
Yogurth (full-fat) gr. 120	200	120	170	245	2	0.1	68	0.7	0.03
Wholemeal bread gr. 50	80	35	6	---	---	1.2	300	0.4	0.08
Jam gr. 10	9	1	1	35	1	0.1	0.7	---	0.01
Beef meat or fish gr. 150	500	300	20	---	---	2	150	---	0.07
Green running beans gr. 300	840	144	100	750	48	3	2	---	0.04
Potatoes gr. 100 (or rusks)	570	54	10	18	15	0.6	7	---	0.04
Mozzarella cheese gr. 70	28	150	403	720	---	0.2	100	4.0	0.05
Eggplants gr. 100	184	33	12	17	5	0.3	26	0.2	0.05
Zucchinis gr. 200s	420	130	42	870	22	0.5	1	0.2	0.08
Lettuce gr. 100	240	31	45	1374	6	0.8	50	0.2	0.05
Spinach gr. 100	531	62	78	2919	54	209	100	0.4	0.07
Carrots gr. 50	120	20	22	3500	2	0.3	25	0.2	0.4
Total values 900 calorie diet	4122	1125	1009	10874	206	12	831	6.4	0.88
Total daily requirement	3100	1000	600/800	4200	60	10/18	2200	7/10	0.8/1
Total values 600 calorie diet	3433	924	736	101.68	153	10.6	461	6.28	0.73

(The rows from Beef meat or fish through Carrots are labelled **600 calories**.)

N.B. Values are expressed in milligrams, except Vit. A in µg (micrograms)

Values of vitamin A are expressed in carotene-B.

Factor of conversion: 1 µg of R:E (retinol equivalent) = 6 µg of B-carotene.

First alternative version of the 900 calorie diet

Breakfast
    1 long, hot and tonic coffee with 2 teaspoons of sweetener[1]

Lunch
    Tagliatelle (or spaghetti or dried beans) g 60 (the weight is intended raw) with peeled tomato g 100, small onions, basil, a teaspoon oil, a pinch of salt when you serve the dish and a teaspoon of grated cheese
    Very lean veal g 150, or grilled lean fish g 150
    Vegetables g 250 (if boiled choose among eggplants, broccoli; if raw, choose among carrots, tomatoes, lettuce seasoned with little oil, oregano and lemon as you like, just a pinch of salt)
    2 rusks g 10 (if you prefer you can eat at breakfast)
    1 coffee (preferably decaffeinated) sweetened with a teaspoon of raw honey g 5

Dinner
    Vegetables (lettuce, zucchini, spinach) cooked or soup, as you like, or consommé g 300-400;
    Very lean veal g 150, or grilled lean fish g 150
    or cheese (fontina, Bel Paese) g 50
    or mozzarella cheese g 30 and 1 hard or soft boiled egg
    with oregano and lemon (only 1 day out of 4);
    2 rusks g 10;
    Fresh fruit g 100 (or stewed string beans g 200-300)

Break at 11 a.m. or afternoon snack at 5 p.m.: low-fat cheese g 100

---

1   We are sorry, but for the time being fruit fancy cakes are sod out! You will find them again when we will repeat the 1200 calorie diet.

Second alternative version of the 900 calorie diet

Breakfast
    1 long, hot and tonic coffee with 2 teaspoons of sweetener

Lunch
    Very lean veal g 150, or grilled lean fish g 150
    Vegetables g 150 (if boiled choose among eggplants, broccoli; if raw, choose among carrots, tomatoes, lettuce seasoned with little oil, oregano and lemon as you like, just a pinch of salt)
    2 rusks g 10
    1 coffee (preferably decaffeinated) sweetened with a teaspoon of raw honey g 5

Dinner
    Soup with pasta or beans or rice or lentils g 50 (together with 300 g of the usual cooked vegetables: lettuce, zucchini, spinach)
    Very lean veal g 150, or grilled lean fish g 150
    or cheese (fontina, Bel Paese) g 50
    or mozzarella cheese g 30 and 1 hard or soft boiled egg
    with oregano and lemon (only 1 day out of 4);
    2 rusks g 10 (if you prefer you can eat at breakfast)
    Fresh fruit g 100 (or stewed string beans g 200-300)

Break at 11 a.m. or afternoon snack at 5 p.m.: low-fat cheese g 100
<u>Piece of advice</u>: (not compulsory, only if you want to favor a greater intake of proteins which provoke antibodies production against infections diseases)

    I day: lunch: meat / evening: grilled fish
    II day: lunch: fish / evening: 1 egg + 30 g mozzarella cheese
    III day: lunch: fish / evening: meat
    IV day: lunch: meat / evening: cheese
    2 evenings out of 4 fruit and 2 evenings out of 4 stewed string beans g 200 (you can match food according to your taste).

Alternative version with a sandwich for lunch (in total about 950 calories) suitable for employees and for those who cannot cook at home and are in a great hurry.

A further possibility of 900 calories diet: "anti-hunger" diet for those who are in a hurry and don't have the time to cook at noon (employees, and so on)

Morning: 8 o'clock Breakfast (80 calories)	1 coffee with a teaspoon sugar milk flakes g 80 - 100
11 o' clock Snack (200 calories)	1 bun or 1 small tart (about g 40) 1 American coffee

You can swap breakfast with snack

13 o' clock Lunch (400 calories)	1 roll 70 g, with 100 g very lean meat (i.e. roast-beef) or alternatively mozzarella cheese g 50 1 teaspoon oil Lemon, some tomato slices and green leaves
20 o'clock Dinner (250 calories)	boiled vegetables, little salt (better no salt to have a diuretic effect) preferably: zucchini, onions, carrots, or: spinach, green string beans seasoned with lemon, vinegar 400 g in total. Fish 100-150. Bread sticks g 22 (2 bags of 10-11 g each) or a slice of bread 30 g

Warning: cholesterol content (max) = about 180 mg

Menu of the 600 calorie diet

Breakfast
  1 coffee sweetened with 10 g of raw honey (or sugar, if you do not like honey)

Lunch
  Lean veal g 150, or grilled lean fish g 150
  Vegetables g 200-300 (if boiled choose among eggplants, broccoli; if raw,
  choose among carrots, tomatoes, seasoned with little oil, oregano and lemon as you like, just a pinch of salt)
  2 rusks g 10
  1 coffee (preferably decaffeinated) sweetened with a teaspoon of raw honey

Dinner
  Vegetables (lettuce, zucchini, spinach) cooked or soup,
  as you like, or consommé g 300-400;
  Lean veal g 150, or grilled lean fish g 150
  or low-fat cheese with milk flakes g 10
  or mozzarella cheese g 30 and 1 hard or soft boiled egg
  with oregano and lemon (only 1 day out of 4);
  2 rusks g 10;
  Fresh fruit g 100 (or stewed string beans g 200-300)

This 600 calorie diet comes from the preceding one (900) but does not include breakfast (except coffee with honey and sugar).

For this diet we can also apply the scheme recommended for the menu and the alternative versions of the 900 calorie diet.

In the column of proteins, the values in brackets refer to the choice of meat / fish in the evening, richer in proteins than the other combinations.

Logical analysis of the chemical composition of the 600 calorie diet

Food and quantity (in gram)	Calories	Proteins (in gram)	Carbohydrates (in gram)	Fats (in gram)	Cholesterol (in mg)
Honey g 15	48	—	12	—	
Meat or fish g 150	135	31	—	1.2	100
Fruit g 100 (apples)	48	0.3	11	0.3	
Rusks g 20	76	2.26	16.6	0.12	
Cow mozzarella cheese g 70 [Meat or fish g 150]	172	13.45 [31]*	0.4	13	66.5
Eggplants g 200	32	2.2	5.2	0.2	
Zucchini g 200	22	2.6	2.6	0.2	
Lettuce g 100	20	1.8	2.2	0.4	
Spinach g 100	31	3.4	2.8	0.7	
Carrots g 50	19	0.57	3.8	0.15	
Total grams		[76]* - 57	56.6	16.27	166.5
Daily total calories	603	203.32 (g 57.58x4 cal)	226.4 (g 56.6x4 cal)	146.43 (g 16.27x9 cal)	
Percentages (optimized)	100%	38.2%	37.5%	24.28%	

Alternative 600 calorie diets

These two diets are a perfect example of a Mediterranean diet and can substitute the standard one for one or the total 10 days.

To raise the calories from 600 to 700, it is necessary to add, daily, 100 g roast-beef or very lean veal or chicken breast. If this food is already included, you can double it (100+100).

The two days which include the egg (main menu and second alternative version) must be followed each every 4 days.

First alternative version of the 600 calorie diet

Breakfast
 1 light coffee
 Skimmed milk g 200

Lunch
 Stewed sole (or salmon) g 200
 Bread g 20 or a bag of bread sticks g 12
 1 orange or a grapefruit g 100

Dinner
 Roasted or stewed chicken breast g 100
 Stewed green string beans g 200
 1 apple g 100
 1 rusk

Second alternative version of the 600 calorie diet

Breakfast
 1 coffee
 Skimmed milk g 200

Lunch
 Spaghetti or tagliatelle g 50 Butter g 10
 1 tablespoon parmesan
 Grilled veal g 100 with lemon and parsley
 1 rusk

Dinner
 Vegetable soup with tomatoes, zucchini, onions g 200-300
 Boiled fish g 200
 Bread g 20 or 2 rusks or 1 bag of bread g 12

Remark about the 600 calories level

As you see, until the last minute of this dietetic program we can speak still of spaghetti (or tagliatelle), of abundant portions of fish, veal, bread and some rusks.

Take comfort from the fact that most people in the world follow a slimming diet which starts immediately with this level of calories. At least, you have reached this stage after 40 days of richer diets!

Milk shakes and nonalcoholic long drinks

American-style shake

The juice of ½ orange, ½ lemon, 1 fruit as you like 100 g, 1 teaspoon sugar. Put all the ingredients into the mixer and mix for about two minutes. Serve immediately.

Orange cocktail or cocktail rosé

Put ½ orange, ½ lemon, 100 g carrots and mix for about two minutes. Add 1 pinch of salt, pepper, 1 ice cube.

Grapefruit cocktail

For six people: 4 grapefruits, 1 orange squeezed, ½ liter mineral water, ice cubes. Serve in chilled glasses with sugared brims.

Flavored hot tea

For six people: 2 oranges, ½ lemon, sugar peel of ½ lemon. After you make tea according to the classical rules, pour the citrus juice into the pot, the peel and sugar.

Cold strawberry and raspberry tea

After you make tea according to the classical rules, let 150 g strawberries wrapped in a clean linen cloth soak for 10 minutes. Remove them and add, if possible, 1 teaspoon of strawberry syrup and 1 of sour black cherry. Water down to big glasses of water, add ice and serve.

Strawberry milk shake

For one person: put into the mixer 100 g strawberry, add 2 teaspoons sugar and 1 glass of skimmed milk. Mix for about two minutes. Serve very fresh.

FIFTH PART

A GOOD EXAMPLE OF THE "HEALTHY DIET" EVEN FOR THOSE WHO DO NOT HAVE TO LOSE WEIGHT

A healthy diet, which can contrast the rise of cholesterol and arteriosclerosis, as well as, important diseases

As it happens for all true and natural things, at a glance you understand, straight away, what there is to understand, without any circumlocutions.

I am pretty sure that my readers have already acquired, at the end of this book, a competence to judge. Certainly, you have more competence than before starting to read this text. But even an incompetent person would understand that the health diet I propose is the only, practicable, long-term diet. Generally speaking, we can say that this sort of food is obvious, almost necessary and irreplaceable, apart from some personal adjustments as to total calories[1].

Of course, yesterday you were invited and for lunch you had meat sauce, cooked in a delicious way (later a brick on you tummy). Of course, today, in the afternoon, you bit into a big piece of nougat left from an old Christmas gift box.

Tomorrow, you are pretty sure, you will tuck into some meat roll, with plenty of pepper and salt, along with more and more dishes, during a banquet you were invited to. That is grand. And the day after tomorrow? And next week? And the other one? What do you want to do, just going on eating like this, starting your old-age at 50? Or reaching 70 years old in perfect shape? If you made up your mind for the last hypothesis, then you can do without the "health diet", which is detoxifying, nourishing and rich in vitamins able to counteract free radicals responsible for cancers, too.

I have created this diet as a frank alternative to another one, invented by some colleagues of mine an afternoon of some years ago. I was taking part in a congress on obesity while I noticed a group of experts from a university in northern Italy. They had created a diet of 1700 calories, that at first glance, seemed a 700 calorie one.

---

1   For men of about 78-85 kg the "Health Diet", in the long run, would result progressively a slimming one and should be raised by adding some more starchy food and proteins (meat and fish).

After a while you could notice that there were many calories, but frankly it seemed that was purposely done to give that impression.

One of the most important points of my diet is the afternoon snack. It is the same as a very decent dinner, but this last one has to be still eaten. And the almost 300 gr of daily starchy food between pasta and bread? And cheese, eggs? And the daily ration of fruit, almost 500 grams? Well, let us examine it together. Firstly its menu, then a per cent and logical analysis, as we have done for the slimming diets of the Progressive Method.

Ideal diet, complete with nutritional factors, vitamins and mineral salts necessary for a correct working of your body. Total: about 2000 calories (by summing up all meals)

Basic food and possible substitutions	Calories
Breakfast	
	65
Full fat milk (also with coffee) g 100 (or 1 jar of full-fat yogurt)	
	72/156
4 rusks (or 60 g bread from the afternoon snack)	
sugar or honey g 15 (3 teaspoons)	48
1 coffee (long, hot, American style, tonic)	--
Total calories	185/268

it follows

Basic food and possible substitutions	Calories
<u>Lunch</u>	
Rice g 60 (or spaghetti) + lentils g 30	227 + 80
Peeled tomatoes, boiled small onions, chilli to season pasta or rice and lentils	----
Roasted chicken breast g 100, with no salt and no other ingredient (or turkey or rabbit)	96
Raw or cooked carrots g 200 + lettuce gr. 100	60
2 teaspoons of olive oil g 10	90
Lemon to season as you like (or balsamic vinegar 2 teaspoons)	—
Bread g 60	156
Fruit as you like g 150 (oranges, apricots, grapes and persimmon)	60
Total calories	769
<u>Afternoon snack</u>	
1 jar of full-fat yogurt	65
Bread g 60 (or eventually the rusks from breakfast)	72/156
Fruit as you like 150 g (or 1 hardboiled egg 1 each 4 days)	60/70
Total calories	210/290

it follows

The afternoon snack is the movable element of this diet. For those people who are used to have a large breakfast, bread eaten in the morning could give more energy and satiety while the rusks (4) eaten in the afternoon could be meant as a dessert together with yogurt spread on them and the fruit. If, vice versa, your problem is not the morning but the evening, my advice is not to split the afternoon snack too much or abolish it completely (as it may happen for want of time). If you eat it at the right time, you are sure not to be too hungry for dinner. In any case you have to eat all its components within 24 hours, even if you abolish it.

An ideal alternative to the fruit of the afternoon snack could be a hardboiled egg. It has almost the same quantity of calories (60↔76) and can be eaten also in the morning (especially if is soft-boiled). It is wrong to think that this food is harmful for the liver if eaten often. The egg contains albumin (the protein of albumen) and some vitamins contained in yolk that a sick liver could not synthesize by itself. The prejudice does exist because its assumption, in subject suffering from stones in the cholecyst, can provoke pains in the abdomen due to contractions of the bile sac. In any case (high cholesterol level), its introduction into the afternoon snack or the breakfast must not exceed one day every 3-4.

Basic food and possible substitutions	Calories
Dinner Bean soup g 40 (dried beans) and boiled vegetables g 200 2 teaspoons of olive oil g 10 (add lemon or balsamic vinegar) Very lean veal or roasted fish g 200, on alternate evenings Bread g 60 Boiled vegetables (zucchini, fennel etc.) g 300 – or raw Fruit as you like g 150 (grapefruit, pineapple, banana) *Total calories*	130 40 90 190 156 60 60 726
Total daily calories (any combination)	**about 2000**

In order to reach 1600 calories our advice is to reduce the bread to 40 g a meal, halve the meat or the evening fish and also the beans from dinner (saving on total calories = 300), and fruit from lunch (60 calories). This is well replaced, as to fibers and minerals, with the huge portion of cooked and raw vegetables, accompaniment to chicken breast (1998 calories – 360 calories = about 1638 calories).

This reduction must be preferred to the abolition of the afternoon snack, which is however rich enough (roll, yogurt, fruit) and has a very important task, that is to reduce the evening hunger, your worst ENEMY!!!

We remind you, however, that this diet is not intended as a slimming one, but just enough to lighten a heavy body. Later, its task will be to keep your body light, healthy, well provided with antitoxins and always ready to spring. In addition, by ensuring a high degree of satiety, it will avoid the risk to eat until you are fit to burst.

The "healthy diet" is a classic example of Mediterranean diet. As you know, this kind of diet is tied to the highest average of human survival.

It contains all known factors (and probably some unknown) which supply our body with all most important minerals (iron, potassium, zinc, magnesium, copper, mini elements such as nickel, cobalt, etc) in a natural way. Moreover, it also contains selenium and all the most important hydro and lip soluble vitamins, especially those with antioxidant functions, that is, antiageing, and therefore above all anticancer. This, thanks to its various natural fibers, plentiful fruits, vegetables, starchy food and pulses. The percentage is optimal too (bread g 120, starchy food and pulses g 160, fruit g 450, vegetables g 650) and in addition it contains few lipids.

Logical analysis of "healthy diet"

Food and quantity (in gram)	Calories (in gram)	Proteins (in gram)	Fats (in gram)	Carbohydrates (in gram)	Cholesterol (in mg)
Full fat milk g 200 (or two jars of full-fat yogurt 100 g each)	130	7	7	9.6	20
Sugar or honey g15	48	---	—	12	
4 rusks	72	2,26	0.12	16.5	
Spaghetti or tagliatelle g 70	257	7,6	0.36	5.5	
Lentils g 30	80	6,2	1.6	12.2	
Tomatoes g 150	20	1	---	3.75	
Chicken breast g 100	96	22,2	0.9	---	68
Carrots g 200	70	2,3	---	15.6	
Oil g 20	180	—	18	---	
Bread g 180 (total)	470	16,2	0.78	100	
Fruit 450 g (total)	192	1,3	1.65	42.7	
Veal or fish g 200 (alternate evenings)	190	40	5	---	140
Beans g 40 (or boiled potatoes g 150)	130	3	0.3	28	
Vegetables g 500 (total)	58-90	9	2	10	
Total grams	—	**114**	**38**	**302**	**228**
Total calories	**2000** (about)	**458** (g 104x4 cal)	**336** (g 50. 50x9 cal)	**1208** (g 282x4 cal)	
Percentages (optimized)	**100%**	**22%**	**16.8%**	**60.4%**	

Data in this scheme and the following have been extracted from various sources, and finally, doing a mean of values, adapted by the Author.

Health diet	K	P	Ca	Vit. A Mg of carotene B	Vit. C Mg of carotene B	Fe	Na	Zn	Vit. B1
Yogurt (full-fat) 2 jars	400	240	340	540	2	0.1	68	0.7	0.03
Spaghetti or tagliatelle gr. 70	200	120	12	---	---	1	20	1.3	0.14
Lentils gr. 30	250	120	50	60	3	4	33	1.1	0.2
Tomato (green) gr. 100	310	25	9	810	25	0.3	7	Tr	Tr
Chicken breast gr. 100	325	214	10	---	---	---	67	0.7	0.08
Carrots gr. 200	480	80	88	14000	8	1.4	100	0.8	0.08
Bread (rolls) gr. 180	300	200	110	0	0	1.3	1400	1.5	0.08
Veal or fish gr. 200	700	350	22	---	---	4.6	200	---	0.4
Dried beans gr. 40	514	Not perc.	60	10	Not perc.	3	227	1.2	0.4
I° total	**3479**	**1300**	**701**	**15420**	**38**	**15.7**	**2122**	**7.1**	**0.8**
Lettuce gr. 100	240	31	45	1374	6	0.8	50	0.2	0.05
Eggplants gr. 100	184	33	12	12	17	03	26	0.2	0.05
Turnip leaves gr. 100	200	49	169	1800	81	2.7	---	---	0.04
Endive gr. 100	380	31	93	1281	35	1.7	10	0.4	0.05
Green tomatoes gr. 100	310	25	9	810	25	0.3	7	Tr	Tr
Apricots gr. 100	320	16	16	2160	13	0.5	---	---	0.03
Orange gr. 100	200	8	12	59	60	0.4	2	0.1	0.03
Persimmons gr. 100	87	16	8	1422	23	0.3	25	0.1	0.02
Pineapple gr. 100	220	8	12	59	60	0.4	2	0.1	0.03
II° general total	**56020**	**1580**	**1115**	**24770**	**348**	**23**	**2242**	**8.2**	**1.31**
Daily requirement	3100	1000	800	4200	60	10/18	2200	7/10	0.8/1

Remarks about the "healthy diet"

We can state that the diet I am proposing, in short, can be followed by:

- who are going to follow the Progressive Method of 2000 and 1600 calories; they can find them ready to use instead of elaborating them by themselves;
- who wants to observe for a given time a caloric level a little bit lower than the normal 2500-2700 calories because he has overeaten (almost always meals are washed down with abundant quantity of alcohol). In this case, 10-15 days on diet are enough to gain a good shape;
- who is not ready from a psychological point of view (or for various reasons) to face all the stages of the Progressive Method and wants to stop at the first detoxifying stage. This is a way to lose 3-4 kg in a month easily, and make weight stable.

Let me venture a remark: if the excess kilos are too many, you miss a great opportunity to stop at the first stage, especially if you reach this one without any difficulty. As I have already said before, the Progressive Method, unique diet in the world with the gradual drop of calories, does not provoke an excessive appetite in the subjects who follow it and allows to reach the last stage without never feeling the classic pangs of hunger. Why then, not continuing with the other diets of the Progressive Method?

Practically, it is the same as going up the steps of a well-planned stair. You can sometimes go up 4-5-6 steps without any effort; on the contrary, it may happen that if the steps do not suit our pace, it is enough to go up a flight to feel tired.

In addition, a field where this diet can be applicable is in the childish and adolescent obesity. Let see together why.

The golden rules of the dietetics foresee about 2000 daily calories for both sexes aged from 6 to 10. You should not be stupefied by the high value of calories in such so young subjects, as since their birth until 18 years old the course is on the way down.

The per cent distribution of 2000 calories in question is very close to that of "healthy diet":

Diet recommended for people of either sex aged 7-11 years (about 2000 daily calories)		"Healthy diet" (about calories) 2000 daily	
proteins	16%	proteins	20%
lipids	28%	lipids	23%
Carbohydrates	56%	Carbohydrates	57%

Remark: it is very clear that, for a child aged 6-10 who starts showing signs of metabolic slackening, is not possible (rightly) already at that age to lower the daily calories, because in full development. In this case, it is already wise to increase the percentage of proteins to detriment of fats, condition besides present in the "healthy diet".

In the following range of age we can find:

Diet recommended for people of either sex aged 12-14 years (about 2500 daily calories)		"Healthy diet" (about calories) 2000 daily	
proteins	16%	proteins	20%
lipids	25%	lipids	23%
Carbohydrates	58%	Carbohydrates	57%

Remark: considered that the adolescent age allows, or better imposes, a dietetic intervention on a overweight subject, a slight reduction of 500 daily calories can reestablish the situation without any sacrifice from the young patient. Once again, the "healthy diet" as it is, without changing a comma, a number, it reveals itself as the most adequate, closest solution to the childish obesity. How is it possible? Is it a pure coincidence? No, it is not. The reason is that this diet is child of good clinical sense, the best virtue, perhaps, for a physician.

Why actors and top models do lose weight in a bad way

Probably because they are people leading a stressing, obsessive, phobic, very similar to a nightmare. I can guarantee to know these people enough and to be familiar with the television world, for my various appearances on the small screen.

Days for these people have a frantic rhythm: in the morning they arrange an engagement or a very important meeting for their career. After two hours, for example, it may happen that the contract fades; two hours later a similar piece of news, and then again after a couple of hours the first hypothesis comes back. At seven o'clock p.m. both possibilities wane and a new one pushes its way. This one will draw the attention during the night, the day after and so on. The people concerned live in a perennial limbo, eating the first food they find (fruit, chips, ice creams, sweets) or refusing food for days, during which they just drink mineral water, grapefruit juice, tea, sugar or presumed detoxifying infusion (in general, even if they declare to the dietician that they eat much pasta or huge steak, this is rarely true).

The lack of the protein minimum makes the facial muscles flabby because of protein release which composes the connective tissue stroma and the wrinkling of the neck lines for the sudden use from the body of collagen and all supporting tissues.

If they do not introduce carbohydrates, lipids and above all proteins, all the noble functions of the organism are alerted and the body, which must elaborate the enzymatic processes, must create immune antibodies (proteins). These last ones are also used to protect itself, and when the supplies are used up, it manages on its own and uses the proteins from muscles, causing legs to be often threadlike.

Practically, people with no problem of time and money to take care of their body and keep it fit, drift along, relieving on food a series of personal problems. So far not *very* much surprises us. On the contrary, what should be blamed with no excuse is the demand to revive their own body rather than from the inside, with a diet, with stupid things, such as "revitalizing massages" which most of the times causes only the breaking of capillary vessels; seaweed compress, often rather exciting for the nervous system and causing allergies and so on. Only beauticians do their job well in these cases (and good business) managing in few hours to restyle only the make-up... pardon me, the face to be precise!

The problem of the daily protein minimum is growing and is becoming more and more a real problem. In fact, an organism should intake, during 24 hours, from 0.8 to 1 gram of proteins per kilo of body weight, a value to be increased during all those illnesses which try our body sorely (infectious disease, or provoking a greater wear for our organism, as hepatic disease).

Well, most people (and those who consider themselves experts fail, too) think that 100 g meat is enough to satisfy this need, while on the contrary, by counting, you can find out that 100 g meat contain only 20 g proteins. Where is it possible to find 50 g more for an average man weighing 70-80 kg?

To start with, let increase meat from 100 to 200 g (or fish is the same). We have reached therefore 40 g. We need 30-40 g more. Starchy foods lend us a precious hand (and indispensable, considered that animal proteins must not be more than 1/3), 100 g bread contain about 7 g; 100 g rice about 7; 100 g potatoes about 2 g. We add therefore 200 g bread and 10 g rice (or pasta) to 200 g meat (or fish) and we will have in total 65 g proteins. Let us introduce, for example, 50 g cheese, which will provide with about 12-14 g proteins (as many fats!)

Very well. We can do this, however, with people eating normally and are not on a diet. Moreover, if you just reflect for a while, it is not so easy to find people which eat all this food daily!

Let summarize:
g 200 meat or fish
g 200 bread
g 100 rice or pasta (or g 150 dried beans or lentils)
g 50 cheese

Why is it not so easy?

A first answer is that generally we are biased towards the meat on the market (cholesterol or other fears as to red meat; chicken meat seems to contain great amounts of estrogens, rabbit cannot be found easily, not to mention pork).

As to fish, there is not any problem apart from the fact that it is too expensive and it is difficult to clean. The frozen one looks suspicious because of preservatives.

People often ignore bread because they think it is too fattening, as well as pasta or rice. It is very difficult to find people eating the above-mentioned quantity daily or globally. Perhaps among these people we can find heavy eaters of ice-creams, puddings, sweets which undoubtedly contain also a high percentage of proteins, but they cannot be taken into consideration to solve the problem of a correct protein minimum.

The same applies to cheese: if you ate 200-300 g a day, rather than 50 g, the problem would be solved (as to numbers) but the values of cholesterol and triglycerides would rocket. In fact, you would eat about 100 g animal fats daily and from the same source: 35 g fats from 100 g cheese, not to mention intestinal irritation and digestive overload.

if the problem cannot be easily solved for a normal daily diet, think about those who follow a low-calorie diet.

When you start a low-calorie diet and you want to rely on the protein minimum, first of all you find yourself in front of the first rule. If fats can be avoided for a short period almost completely, the same does not apply to carbohydrates. Therefore the protein minimum is hardly reducible because the greater reductions can be carried out exactly on the other two groups of food.

The task to elaborate diets with a lower and lower content of calories becomes therefore more complicated. In fact, if we want to introduce 200 g fish or meat for a normal subject who does not follow any diet, the decision of keeping still an acceptable quantity of starchy food (200 g bread, 100 g rice) and 50 g cheese, provokes a rise in calories. If you include also an indispensable (and healthy) contribution of fruit and vegetables, olive oil, pulses, potatoes and so on, we are back again (without doing it purposely, but for a set course) to the caloric levels and percentages of the "Health diet".

This one, through the reasoning of the protein minimum, comes up again as an example hardly surmountable between slimming and detoxifying diets in the long run during which you do not leave anything out. The task to keep the protein minimum by lowering calories is becoming more difficult.

However, as to diets with a more specific caloric level of the Progressive Method, which we have already analyzed in the previous part (1200-900-600-700) well, we can ascertain with great satisfaction that the protein minimum of all of them, elaborated during their writing out, are perfectly compatible with the golden rules of dietetics.

The 1200 calorie level can rely - from Monday to Sunday - on an algebraic average of 70.28 g a day, and in addition on subjects weighing at the beginning 80 (A_1 and 70 kg (A_2). The 900 calorie level, basic intermediate stage, stabilizes on 85 g; as well that of 600 calories with 76 g.

In conclusion, I summarize the main functions carried out by pure organism from the most important types of proteins.

Fundamental biological functions of proteins	
Types of proteins	**Functional principles**
Enzymes	Highly specific catalysts for metabolic reactions
Polipeptic hormones	Regulators of metabolic processes
Protein-nucleus	Transmission of hereditary characters and protein synthesis
Respiratory pigment	Transport of oxygen to tissues
Antibodies	Defense infectious diseases
Carrier factors of various substances and metabolites	Lipids, fat acids, iron, etc..
Contractile proteins (actomyosin)	Muscular contraction
Structural sclero-proteins	Connective tissue, bones, etc.

Any further remark is superfluous, also because this is not the right place to study this topic in depth overmuch.

There is a "poison" which, exonerated by Food and Drug Administration in the USA, can come back to our table

At the beginning of 1984, the Food and Drug Administration established a special unit (Task Force) which was given the task to examine and interpret the recent scientific literature related to sugars, sugars derived from corn and inverted sugar. This special unit, in November 1985, compiled an internal preliminary report where it stated that no conclusive evidence does prove that sugar, eaten at present levels, provokes any danger to people's health.

A diet with a high content of sugar may provoke unwanted effects on glucose tolerance and on metabolism of insulin considering experiments made with heavy administrations.

However, if we consider the present levels of sugar consumption in the USA, there is no persuasive and scientific evidence about the related risks. Sugars are an independent factor of risk if associated to the development of an altered tolerance to glucose (in the USA the consumption of sugars reaches 60 kilos per year and per person; 45 in France and 30 in Italy). "There is no evidence which justifies an alteration to the conclusions of the report from SCOGS in 1976 (Select Committee on GRAS Substances of FASEB). The consumption of sugars is related to diabetes as if it were any non-specific source of energy". In short, it is the same as saying that the consumption of sugars, as to the genesis of diabetes, represents only one of the many components of energy taken from food.

In addition, the report draws some important conclusions, as follow.

We cannot prove that the consumption of sugars is a factor of risks for the lipidemic and lipoprotein aspect in healthy subjects. There is no evidence that proves, in addition, that the present consumption of sugars contributes to the development of hypertension (Doctor Allan L. Forbes)[1].

---

1   Extract from "L'informatore Alimentare. Mensile di Scienza e Cultura dell'Alimentazione", anno VII, Edizioni ENPF, Turin.

Technical section

The importance of local treatment associated to the diet, to fight against localized obesity

Five obese women out of ten present ginoide or matronly-like obesity, in which the fat is accumulated on the hips, on the bottom of thighs and on the knees. Even if it may sound paradoxical, many women in this situation would do it better not to start a diet, because they will surely lose weight more in the upper part, which is not necessary, while the bottom part will lose weight less and less. At last, the figure will be more disproportionate than before.

Let's see why. By cellulitis we mean a particular type of adipose tissue. Because of pathogenic and metabolic causes, which are still unknown, the stroma, that is the fibrous structure supporting the cells, gets thicker and therefore it causes a bigger consistency of adipose accumulations.

The most important consequence is that, because of the fibrous thickening, these areas become less oxygenated than the others. As a result, they get rid of toxins more slowly, triggering a vicious circle more and more, that is a mechanism of cellular degeneration (the exact name of cellulitis is in fact extensive skin lipodystrophy).

These areas, less oxygenated than others (with normal fat), are partially excluded from the changes of metabolism with particular tendency to put on weight before, and, to lose weight after.

A slimming diet, even if followed in an exemplary way, will hardly be able to make patient get rid of localized adipose pads, especially if they are mainly composed from cellulitis.

The way out form this trap is to combine a well balanced diet (that applies to men, too) with a whole series of treatment on the adipose mass so that, the result is not only faster, but much more well-proportioned.

The consequence is that the loss of weight will occur more where it is more necessary (hips, thigh measurement and knees for women and paunch for men).

Moreover, the big advantage of such a combined method will be that, in a lot of cases, it will be enough to lose few kilos to obtain the reduction of a lot of centimeters on several measurements.

The best treatments to use in the therapy of pads and cellulitis are ionophoresis applications, mesotherapy local injections and massage.

The various types of bandaging (pressure therapy) have not any effects on centimeter reduction. Others similar practices compress some parts of the body which expand again, when the action of the instrument finishes.

Similar to what happened with the use of the computer in slimming diets (in spite of the great interest at the beginning) the use of the laser beam in the cellulitis treatment has produced scarce results.

The mesotherapy is the principal treatment in the cellulitis and in the adipose pads.

Using a plate with several tiny needles, it is possible to distribute directly, where necessary, particular medicines' mixtures that break the fibrous barriers of the connective tissue that develop and shut up the fat. These different chemical compositions include also drugs necessary to reactivate the metabolism of these areas and to give back tone even to stretch marks and flabby tissues.

Contrary to what some state, for ignorance or inexperience, the treatment is neither painful at all, nor leave any hematomas, even in those who suffer with varicose veins in the legs.

When these problems occur, it is almost always because the therapy has been practiced by doctors without any specialization in this area, or by beauticians, or even worse, by hairdressers.

Frequently Asked Questions

Question:
Which is the main reason that has lead you to create your Progressive Method?
Why did you think about a "step-like slimming" diet?

Answer:
Around the end of the 70s, the most outstanding idea was the following: if obesity was very severe, you had to follow more drastic diets, the so-called "Shock-diet". As I have already explained in the first chapters of my book, jockeys occasionally follow this much-reduced alimentation (about 400 calories) for a couple of days when they have to lose weight in order to take part in a race. It consists in two steaks and some salad. Nowadays (if still followed) it would be better for your health to replace it with two small sandwiches with roast-beef and some salads. Bread is useful to cover the minimum glycidic quota and not to provoke ketosis, which will later transform into acetonomiae.

Therefore, this caloric level of about 400 calories in an obese patient, especially of masculine sex, soon provokes an extraordinary and striking loss of weight, which makes him lose much weight in few days.

The patient, of course, will inform friends and acquaintances of his loss of weight, also because many of them will notice the change and when they will meet him, they will ask why.

The "news", which today we call the "message", will be born. Many of them will welcome this news without reservations because ignorance makes this event seem miraculous when, on the contrary, it is quite normal. In fact, an obese patient, used to swallow more than 3000 calories a day, can lose much weight in a short time with 400 calories.

Unfortunately, the patient will take again much weight for the following reasons.

There are no further steps down below 400 calories and it is not possible to follow this kind of diet for more than 10-15 days. Therefore, the patient will rise the caloric intake provoking the hectic increase of weight. This situation will be no "message" for anybody. All those people who had received the first message, will be convinced and spread the rumor that eating so little makes possible to lose weight for ever.

On the other side, not all those who always followed the same diet (the so-called balanced diet of about 1200 calories) were able to lose many kilos in the long distance. The reason was that their metabolism seemed to conform to the caloric reduction, which was acceptable, everything considered. This situation, on the other side, created in the patients what I described in my book "the chronicity of a diet".

I had therefore the intuition, around the mid '80s, that the only way to try was to start from an initial caloric level superior to the so-called balanced diet.

For example, in a patient with more than 90 kilos, I thought right to start from 2000 calories, and then going down progressively, to the 600-calorie levels. We have to highlight that the span of time was about two months and not immediately as people did before. Afterwards, having almost reached an ideal weight, I thought to rise again, little by little, for 30 days more through the previous steps, until you reach the initial diet (1600-2000 calories). This itinerary, this dietetic swing was nicknamed "Progressive Method" and the idea was soon patented. The book after a while was published by De Agostini and was patented for The United States too (1987) and Prof. Carlo Sirtori, Nobel Prize candidate, wrote the preface.

Question:

Mr. D'Antoni, which ones are the advantages of the Progressive Method you mention in your book?

Answer:

The Progressive Method is an idea, a slimming scheme, a "dietetic itinerary". I noticed however since the beginning that this dietetic itinerary deserved to be followed by patients. Unlike other diets, there was not the "leap in the dark" of the drastic caloric reduction. In fact, it was tolerated very well and made it possible to follow the most delicate professions such as pilot, air captain, motor racer, surgeons, managers, and so on. In addition to the previous advantages, there was one more. It was becoming increasingly evident during the weight control at different intervals (follow-up) that too many obese patients showed a major resistance to put on weight again after they finished the course and come to normal alimentation. These patients had accepted to follow the Progressive Method, rather than the constant balanced diets.

It was then clear that the dietetic swing had been able to influence somehow the relative maintenance of the new weight reached especially those who had followed the diet in a correct way.

I say relative and not absolute because these people even if under an intensive overalimentation, will put on weight soon or later. I think, for example, to compare it with a medical treatment, a procedure, which would not protect a population completely from getting sick of a certain illness but make the infection spread with more difficulties respect to a sample of non-treated people. This is already very much. Let me say it.

Question:

Mr. D'Antoni, does the original theory that you make glimpse in your book, consist in the discovery of set point?

Answer:

No, not at all. Some northern American authors started speaking of the set point since the 70s. The most important thing, however, is that some scholars, with in-depth studies in the field of obesity, began to suppose that the human being was provided with a programmed regulation point (set-point) for adipose fats. The meaning was that if adipose fats decrease in volume, the organism keeps the anabolic biochemical reactions going. We are speaking from a very general point of view. In my book, this topic is widely dealt with in the chapter "What are the main explanations given until today about the origin of obesity".

If the same adipose deposits, on the other hand, increase in thickness, the set point works well and succeeds in blocking their further formation. Little by little, the concept of set point has lost its initial meaning and has become, for greater convenience, synonym of regulating center. Its location has been unanimously set in the diencephalic hypothalamus, one of the cerebral regions.

In the past and nowadays too, people speak about "diencephalic obesity" codified even in medical treatises. My scientific remark consists in the facility of obeses to keep the weight stable after having followed the Progressive Method. They find it easier than other patients who have preferred to follow a balanced diet and have not wanted to carry out the proposed drop and rise of calories.

We must suppose that the "dietetic swing" (dietetic itinerary) of the Progressive Method, should succeed in exercising an action of bewilderment and unblock of this hypothalamic cerebral point (set point), thus favoring a better regulating point, more physiological for the future.

Therefore, this drop and rise of calories in obese people works very well. I gave the name of "Theory of the shock of the set point by Mr. M. D'antoni" to this action of the dietetic swing which influence the functioning of the center (see chapter: the theory the Progressive Method is based on). It

137

is obvious that what we have said in very simple words corresponds to more complicated and sophisticated reactions of biochemists today studied by the loftiest minds, whom I invite to make deeper the phenomenon that has been possible to observe and give further scientific explanations.

What we are speaking about deals with neuroendocrinology. Researchers study even the secretion from single groups of the brain neurons.

Question:

I should lose only 5-6 kilos. Is it all right losing them with your method? My job is not heavy, I'm an employee, I work in an office. I am a forty-five-year old woman, I'm 1.63, my weight is 63 kg. Luckily my weight is not 70 kg as the subject A_2!

Answer:

Generally speaking, I would say if you followed a hypocaloric balanced diet (1200 calories) continually for one month, maybe you would not reach your aim. Moreover it might rise a problem: when you pick up again from 1.200 to a normal alimentation (1800-2000 calories), in this case, it is likely you take again all the kilos lost little by little. <u>In my opinion, it is much better losing weight with the Progressive Method.</u> The "dietetic swing" is very good for your set-point. It is like an exercise, which keeps this mechanism always efficient. In this case, for example, you might use the following dietetics planning:

HOW TO LOSE 5 KILOS IN THIS CASE

Descending phase of calories:

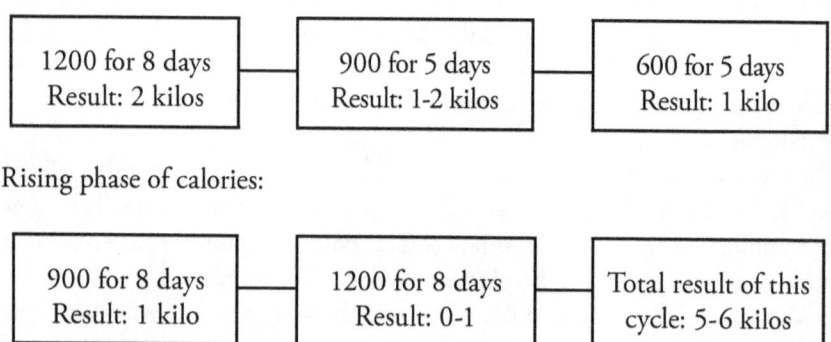

1200 for 8 days Result: 2 kilos	900 for 5 days Result: 1-2 kilos	600 for 5 days Result: 1 kilo

Rising phase of calories:

900 for 8 days Result: 1 kilo	1200 for 8 days Result: 0-1	Total result of this cycle: 5-6 kilos

Final diet: 1800-2000 according to the sex and daily type of effort

Question:

You say in your book that some physical activity is important and that your set-point works better in the future, especially after reaching the ideal weight. What kind of activity and how much time do you have to spend on it?

Answer:

One or two hours a week are good enough. If you have no time to go to the gym, it will be sufficient to go for a brisk walk just for two hours a week. In our ancestral past, men too, like animals, walk a lot to get their food.

Question:

Say I do not lose all the kilos of a given step, during the dropping of calories in the Progressive Method. Is it better to follow for some days the same level of calories, or going to the next step?

Answer:

If this happens in the first steps of the descending phase, it is better to prolong for 7-8 days the step you were following. If vice versa, this happens in the last steps of the descending phase, then it is necessary to follow at once the inferior step or rising again so that you do not linger too much over the low-calorie periods. This is not because situations of lack can take place or have already happened, but for an excess of prudence.

Question:

Is it possible that in medicine it does not exist an absolute reference point as to the right time for each loss of weight? No book gives an answer.

Answer:

This is true. The explanation lies in the fact that each loss of weight has to be considered in the overall point of view of the patient. My book has been the first in the world to deal with the revelation of this "Mystery". In the chapter "There are criteria and precise rules to judge a slimming cycle satisfactory", I have created a sort of equation. On one side, there is the number of kilos lost, on the other, the way you lose them. Each element has to be in an optimal relationship with all the other factors. For example, what is the point of losing ten kilos in a month (supposing this is possible) if you have been fasting for all the time?

On the contrary, what is the point of being satisfied with having lost 10 kilos in a year, putting forward of having done few sacrifices. On the other side you had to follow anyway a diet, you had to weigh food and so on.

Question:

Would it be better instead of speaking of slimming cycle, to propose a very slow loss of weight little by little, too?

Answer:

Unfortunately this option would be valid, but on the contrary it is not so. In this case you do not put 5 dollars a day into a moneybox and you find 1800 at the end of the year. Things are completely different and only professional people like me, used to live in a tight spot with obese people, know why! In everybody's life, there are different moments. The time you have to study for a competitive examination, to learn how to play bridge, to learn how to use a computer, to learn how to play sports. There is also the right time you deserve to follow a slimming diet. It must be like this because the period dedicated to slimming very often might be crossed by personal or familiar events. If some of them are particularly important, most of the time they induce to interrupt your diet. I might quote uncountable statistics which have been elaborated in my office regarding some slimming diets which have been interrupted for different reasons. All of them were important reasons and only few cycles have been taken up again with the same commitment. Among these – and here lies my answer – the diets taken up again were those which had reached at least the half part of the Progressive Method.

Question:

In recent time, you hear of "reasonable" weight. What is this?

Answer:

Some authors say that is enough to lose also few kilos (until 6-7 in a patient weighing 100 kilos) which make the patients feel lighter and dynamic, in this way, patients improve the tendency to diabetes and other disease of exchange (hyperuricemia, hypertension, and so on).

For obese people this would mean, in my opinion, an unconditional surrender. All the more reason, for the great number of successful patients that I have followed for many years, it is like saying it is not worthy to put aside much money because maybe later you will spend it again. It is much better to put aside just little money to have some constant cash. But when what you set aside is little, it is not very often "well protected", I mean that on the first occasion you can spend your small sacrifice!

Question:
What does behavioral therapy of obesity mean? Why don't you deal with it in your book?

Answer:
Behavioural therapy means that, since patients put on weight because of wrong alimentary behaviours, you must focus on these ones and not on diets.

I tried myself too in my office to include a psychologist during the slimming diet.

If the psychologist is very good, he will be able to stir up in the muddle of consciousness and unconsciousness of each patient. Existential conflicts, disappointments, frustrations, anxiety will emerge and will make slimming slide in second, third, fourth place!! Obese people often look for a good alibi not to lose weight.

Personally, I never needed to recur to this kind of therapy.

I have always been acknowledged great spirit of communication.

Most patients have always shown optimism, spirit of initiative, efficiency, and never passiveness.

In conclusion, I repeat again the saying you can read at the beginning of my book: "Obesity is not a sweet cradle, vice versa a crambling alcove you can go out from with intelligence, shrewdness and will".

Question:
Speaking about the different types of meat, you recommend to use roast beef as lean meat. Some people don't like it, for example, I don't. Which other kind of veal meat do you recommend?

Answer:
For example, the meat from the young veal (so-called milk veal from the Italian language). It contains only 1-2% of fats each 100 grams. You can also choose chicken breast (white meat only). Alternatively, rabbit meat which is very lean in Italy, like horse and turkey. Of course, beef is very tasty, but in some cases it contains the same quantity of fats as pork (18%). I take the opportunity to outline that cooked and raw ham contain many fats we cannot eliminate because they are mixed tightly with the lean part (about 38%).

Question: are all the listed food quantities to be meant cooked or uncooked? I didn't notice this was specified in your book.

<u>Answer:</u> actually, you are right. As a matter of fact, we have not specified we use the food uncooked since this is automatic during any correct diet. In fact, according to the length and the way of cooking, food can intake enormous quantities of water. They can even weigh 4 times more than the original weight. I will never forget a particular event. It was late (about 1 or 2 a.m.) and a diabetic patient of mine phoned me. He had lost his weight, he was following a diet of maintenance and he ate a whole tub of rice without complaining of any disease. Since he had ordered the same for one member of his family, when he weighed this one, he had the unpleasant surprise to notice a weight of 800 grams! He was terrified by the idea of having eaten that quantity. There and then I advise him in any case to take an additional tablet of his drug against diabetes and to keep calm. The following day the chef of the restaurant where he had bought the rice, told him that the maximum uncooked quantity could not be more than 150 grams!! This reveals a lot about the quantity of cooked or uncooked food. Who prescribes "cooked" quantity, generally makes a good impression but takes away food from the patient!!

<u>Question:</u> what are the most frequent complications of obesity?

<u>Answer:</u> they are many, and all of them are serious enough. It is a topic I didn't speak much about because it is very long to complete it and generally, in diet books, together with the description of vitamins and compositions of food, they are included to make the book 50 pages longer. Since our goal is that to lose weight and not to bear the consequences of obesity (at least, we do hope it!) for the time being I only will analyze it later.

<u>Question:</u> what is the percentage of obesity today in Italy and n the USA?

<u>Answer:</u> according to the multi-purpose survey of ISTAT (Italian Institute of Statistics), the 6.9% of Italians in 1990-1991 suffered from "serious" obesity. According to a most updated survey from the same ISTAT in the years 1997-1998 such percentage was rising to about 9%. In the USA it is raising more and more, astronomically. It is the second prevented factor of death-risk. An epidemic which absorbs the 10% of the health spending. In addition "II Giornale del Medico" informs us that in Italy (besides the 9-10% of obeses) a man out of two and a woman out of three are overweight. In the USA the percentages would speak about 1/3 of the adult obese population and 1/4 of teenagers.

<u>Question:</u> dr. D'Antoni, since we are all "obliged" continuously to eat out, either for work problems or for being invited or for our free-time (weekends)

which one is the strategy we have to follow not to lose all the results achieved so far? This problem is particularly serious during the periods in which the different subjects of the various types have to follow the weeks with low-calorie intakes.

<u>Answer:</u> Anyway, the problem does exist and it is not very easy to solve. We can try together, recurring to the so-called "common sense" which today is very hard to find. If you go to the restaurant, to conform with the others (remember that today it represents the most important thing as to your image), you'd better have rather than the first course (this is very common in Italy and it is always based on pasta, rice, tagliatelle with a lot of seasoning, oil and salt), two big oysters which contain few calories, or a starter.

This may sound a little bit snobbish but the content in calories will be less (generally you can have salads with chunks of chicken or fish). Apart from the limit case, I give you a couple of examples which I consider personally tasty: ham and white melon (even if you can eat more melon than ham and makes you angry to leave ham in your plate!). You can have smoked salmon seasoned with oil and lemon, laid on well buttered crunchy canapé but leave out the butter and canapé and have only the dripped salmon. Then you can try the starters based on croquettes and chips (personally, they don't lead me into temptation and I could leave them in my plate without tasting them). You could do with the prawn cocktail with sauce. At the end, the calories are the same of a first course in this case, too. Try anyway to avoid the cocktail sauce. If you choose the second course, you can have lean veal or chicken breast, or turkey, roasted, (big portions anyway). I warn you to speak with the maitre and tell him to cook it without oil and salt. Point out that you would like to have the grill cleaned not to absorb all the oil cooked and the salt from the food cooked before yours. On the contrary, you can complain and pretend they cook again your meat or fish. When it is served, ask for some green leaves, some tomatoes, then season with few drops of oil and plenty of lemon. You can have a couple of bread-sticks. For dessert, eat the half of it, don't make anybody understand you are on diet and tell everybody you don't like sweets that much. You will drink a drop of dessert wine. And your meal is over.

Let's count the calories introduced: 2 oysters or a salad with chunks of ish or chicken dripped under hal lemon: about 100-150. Very lean veal or roast-beef or a slice of roasted fish (even if azure fish - 150 gr. in all the cases) = no more than 250-300 calories, included the eventual cooked or uncooked green salad. Well, this time you managed to pass the challenging "restaurant" test with a total of 700 calories, included coffee with sweetener at the end (For heaven's sake! You have just finished eating half portion of sweet with cream, which could also be also Saint-Honoré!). It is true, there is also the possibility to ask the waiter for a fruit salad. In this case you should consider the sugar (already contained in fruit) and the eventual syrup made of extrasugar. You'd better avoid it as soon as possible. Much better to have the sweet instead. Some people of your group will soon change their mind about the fact that <u>you are not always on a diet</u>.

If you go to a pizzeria, things are even easier than you might think. There, in fact, you can simply have a pizza. You don't have to face the first problem, that is the starter or the first course; if somebody orders the famous big dish of chips or rice croquette or similar you could say without any problem that you don't eat them because they give you a bloated feeling (which is absolutely true). Then, here is the winning idea. Since even the plainest pizza (tomato and mozzarella cheese) contains about 1200 calories, instead of eating only half (making a fool of yourself) you, old fox, will order lean meat or fish, like in a restaurant (without oil, salt, etc.). You will tell the others that you do like pizza but only as a starter and it doesn't fill you up. In this case you won't feel in a condition of psychological inferiority but on the contrary your position will turn prestigious and you will make them feel easy-going and easily satisfied. Soon after the pizzas are ready, somebody of your group (it doesn't matter if you are a woman or a man) will think it right to cut a hot and crunchy slice of their pizza and put it in your plate. That will be enough until the waiter will bring you your dish of meat or fish with salad.

The "sweet" - test will not take place (at least in Italy). In pizzeria they serve sweets rarely (like cake or similar). Maybe somebody will ask for a big cup of ice-cream with whipped cream. But you are not obliged to order it, it is not the same as refusing the sweet at the restaurant. For example you can say that you have already eaten two ice-creams so far which does not apply to sweets. Just imagine somebody who, even if he could afford it at 8-9 o'clock p.m. has already eaten two portions of sweet: he would be considered not very sound.

As to buffets, nobody exactly notices what you put into your dish and you can have a wide possibility of choice. The only embarrassing situations are those of dinners at home. You don't have the famous possibility to order lean meat or fish or roasted turkey without oil and salt categorically. Unfortunately when you are invited at home you must put up with pigouts. At restaurant, in fact, nobody puts on weight because portions are always controlled and they follows etiquette.

<u>Question:</u> Dr. D'Antoni, how many calories do a hamburger and a brioche with ice-cream and whipped cream contain?

Answer: I don't know exactly but we can try to find it out: hamburger: minced meat about 100-150 g with a minimum of 20% of fats = 350-400 calories; roll gr 100 = 250 calories. Vice versa (answering another frequent question) the brioche is very fat, it contains 350-400 calories + 200-300 calories for the ice-cream; the same applies for the whipped cream: total = about 1000-1200 calories.

Question: Dr. D'Antoni, how much wine can we drink, or coke or other drinks?

Answer: The role of alcohol seems rather complex. Undoubtedly some salutary effects are proved. For example, abolishing and making antagonist the atherogenic effect of a diet rich in cholesterol. Exerting a certain prevention on cardiovascular disease. Such salutary effects seem however limited to a daily consumption not exceeding 50 grams of alcohol (corresponding to about half a liter of wine).

Some, on the contrary, state that it provokes, sooner or after, especially in predisposed subjects, hepatic fibrosis, that is the hardening of the organ.

When you follow a slimming treatment however it must be banned, since (and this seems proved) even if you drink normal quantities, by eating less food, the alcoholic rare grows more respect the value you have when you eat normally.

Therefore, the danger is that the high concentration, during low-calorie diets, can damage the liver and pancreas. That is the reason why I have always been advised not to allow its use when patients are on a diet, precautionally.

On the other side, it is not so difficult to make patients get out of this habit, even if they have drunk it for many years. Many are those who get used to do without, drinking at its place, some glasses of fizzy drinks. These last ones are so much blamed, only because they contain some gram of sugar and some bubbles!

Anyway my idea is to allow 1-2 little glasses a day of wine of 100 gr. each one – 170 of beer.

As to whiskey (and all spirits) it seems that even some drops in a glass, with a lot of ice, can give a nice feeling. If you still feel thirsty, you can drink all the mineral water in the world, even sparkling. Either bubbles or water, even whole bottles, don't make you put on weight!

Don't forget, in conclusion that my book contains also some particular tea and sophisticated milk-shakes.

Bibliography
For further information

Cabanac, M. Duclaux, R.& Spector, N. H. Sensory feedback regulation of body weight: Is there a ponderostat? Nature, 1971, 229,125-127.

Nisbett. R. Hunger, obesity and the Ventromedial hypotalamus. Psycol. Rev. 79, 433-453, 1972.

Albert Simeons: Chorionic Gonadotrophin in the treatment of obese women. Amer. Journal of Clinical Nutrition 13 -1963 pp. 197-98.

Bray G. A. Gallagher T. F. Manifestations of hypothalamic obesity in man. A comprehensive investigation of eight patients and a review of the literature. Medicine, 1975; 54: 301-30

Le Magren J. Body energy balance and food intake: a neuroendocrine regulatory mechanism - Physiol. Rev. 1983, 63: 315-86

Acheson KJ, Schutz Y, Bessard T et al. Carbohydrate metabolism and de novo lipogenesis in human obesity. Am J Clin Nutr, 1987, 45, 78-85.

Stunkard A.J. - Sorensen T.I.A. - Hanis et al. An Adoption study on human obesity. N. Engl. J. Med. 1986 - 314. 193-8

Mokshangundam M.J., Sheela L, et al. The influence of different methods on basal metabolic rate measurements in Human subjects. Am J Clin Nutr 1989; 50: 731-6

Società Italiana di Nutrizione Umana-LARN (Livelli di Assunzione Giornaliera Raccomandati di Energia e Nutrienti per la popolazione italiana). Roma, 1986-87.

Harris RBS. Role of set point in regulation of body weight. FASEB J 1990; 4: 3310-18

Foster GD, et al. Controlled trial of the metabolic effects of a very low calorie diet. Short and long terms effects. American J Clinical Nutrition 1990: 51: 167-72

Bray G. A. (1992): A survey of the opinions of obesity experts on the causes and treatment of obesity. American Journal of Clinical Nutrition suppl. 1,55: 151S-154S.

PI-SUNYER, FX: The role of very-low calorie diets in obesity. Am J Clin Nutr, 56:240S-3S. 1992

Goldestein D.J. (1992): Beneficial effects of modest weight loss. International Journal of Obesity 16, 397-415

Bosello O., Dalle Grave R., R. Zamboni M., Armenini P. Fisiopatologia e clinica della fluttuazione del peso corporeo: la "Weight cycling syndrome". Obesità '92 Atti XII congresso UICO, 716, 1992

Dalle Grave R. (1994). II peso ragionevole. Che cos'e? Come raggiungerlo, come mantenerlo. Verona, Positive Press.

Pagano R. et al., 1994, Overweight and Obesity in Italy 1990-91, International J. Obesity.

Maria Antonia Fusco; Maria Grazia Carbonelli - Trattamento dietetico dell'obesità - Atti del XIV Congresso dell'Unione Italiana contro l'obesità - La clinica Dietologica - vol. 24 - Fascicoli 1-6; 1997.

Franco Contaldo, Giuseppe Rosato - Terapia dell'obesità; Medico e Metabolismo, Anno 1° n.2, 1997.

Franco Contaldo, A. Esposito - La leptina: proteina che regola il peso corporeo. Medico e Metabolismo 1:79-1997.

To educate to the quality in obesity management Abstracts 16th International Congress of Nutrition. Montreal 1997

Livelli di assunzione Raccomandata di energia e Nutrienti per la popolazione italiana (LARN). Società Italiana di Nutrizione Umana, Revisione 1996.

F. Fidanza: tabelle di composizione dei cibi, Estr. Nutriz. Umana Idelson N. Napoli

Shah M and Garg A. High-far and high carbohydrate diets and energy balance. Diabetes Care, 1996, 19, 1142-1152.

Hellerstein MK. De novo lipogenesis in humans: metabolic and regulatory aspects. Eur J Clin Nutr, 1999, 53 (suppl. 1), S63-S65.

Yves Schutz - Does the conversion to fat contribute to obesity in humans? OBESITY MATTERS -1999, Vol. 2 n. 2, Mediscript limited, London.

Carruba OM, D'Amico B, Falci L, Heymsfield SB, Nisoli E, Pietrobelli A, II trattamento farmacologico nel sovrappeso e nell'obesità 1998 Ediz. Edra.

Patrizia Maria Gatti - L'evoluzione funzionale dell'organo adiposo. Cenesthesi, n. 4, Anno VI, 2000.

Circadian rhythm of hunger sensation in obese patients: Effects of a short term moderately hypocaloric diet with a substitutive med. Tatati - Vendetti -Puxeddu - De Rosa - Coda - De Francesco - De Marco - De Laurentis -Fontana - Cugini - Eating Weight disorders 6: 214 - 219 -2001, Editrice Curtis.

Campfield LA, Smith FJ, Burn P. The OB protein (leptin) pathway - a link between adipose tissue mass and central neural network. Horm Metab Res 1996; 28: 619-32.

Dryeden S, Williams G. The role of hypotalamic peptides in the control of energy balance and body weight Curr Opin Endo Diabets 1996; 3: 51-58

Istituto Nazionale di Ricerca per gli Alimenti e la Nutrizione - Tabelle di composizione degli Alimenti - Aggiornamento 2000 - Edra Medical Publishing - D New Medic.

C.R. Sirtori - Recombinant apolipoproteins come of age Nutr. Metab. -Cardiovascular Dis.(1995) 5: 81-83.

M. Mancini. Metabolismo. Trattato di Fisiopatologia medica. F. Magrassi, vol. III. Soc. Editrice Universo - Napoli.

Verga Salvatore - Buscemi Silvio - Le obesità primitive e secondarie - La Medicina Internazionale n° 8 -1995.

Claudio Marcello Caldarera - Biochimica Sistematica Umana CLUEB, Bologna, 1995.

SIO - Società Italiana per l'Obesità - Newsletter, vol.2. Anno 2001

Thierry Souccar - Règime prehistorique - Science et Avenir, Paris - Mai 2001

Paolo De Cristofaro - Basi metodologiche dell'approccio psiconutrizionale - SEE: Editrice, Firenze 2002

F. Fidanza - The search for the historical roots of the Italian Mediterranean Diet: From antiquity to the first half of XIX century. Diab. Nutr. Metab. 15: 131 - 135, 2002